Manual of PSYCHOSOCIAL NURSING INTERVENTIONS

Promoting Mental Health in Medical-Surgical Settings

Edited by

Susan Lewis, RN, CS, PhD

Psychiatric Nurse Clinical Specialist
Veterans Administration Medical Center
Louisville, Kentucky

Ruth Dailey Knowles Grainger, PhD, ARNP, CS

Nurse Psychotherapist—Private Practice
Miami, Florida

William A. McDowell, PhD

Licensed Psychologist, Professor
Department of Counseling and Rehabilitation
Marshall University
Huntington, West Virginia

Robert J. Gregory, PhD

Senior Lecturer
Department of Psychology
Massey University
Palmerstown North, New Zealand

Roberta L. Messner, RNC, MSN, CIC

Psychiatric Nurse Clinical Specialist
Veterans Administration Medical Center
Huntington, West Virginia

1989

W.B. SAUNDERS COMPANY
Harcourt Brace Jovanovich, Inc.

Philadelphia • London • Toronto • Montreal • Sydney • Tokyo

W. B. SAUNDERS COMPANY
Harcourt Brace Jovanovich, Inc.

The Curtis Center
Independence Square West
Philadelphia, PA 19106-3399

Library of Congress Cataloging-in-Publication Data

Manual of psychosocial nursing interventions.

Includes index.
1. Psychiatric nursing. 2. Nursing—Social aspects.
I. Lewis, Susan.

RC440.M264 1989 610.73′68 89–10306

ISBN 0–7216–5763–X

Editor: Thomas Eoyang
Designer: Joanne Carroll
Production Manager: Peter Faber
Manuscript Editor: Joni Fraser
Indexer: Nancy Newman

Manual of Psychosocial Nursing Interventions:
Promoting Mental Health in Medical-Surgical Settings ISBN 0–7216–5763–X

Printed in the United States of America.

Last digit is the print number: 9 8 7 6 5 4 3 2 1

Oliver Wendell Holmes once commented that some of us die with the music still in us. Indeed, there is music in all of us and to express it is a gratifying experience.

Throughout life we encounter people who encourage us to discover the unique melodies within us. Harmonies are created when we combine our tunes with others to compose symphonies of creativity.

When we combine our creative rhythms with others, it becomes a harmonic symphony. We gratefully dedicate this book to those individuals who have helped us release the music:

Arthur & Novella, Cindy, Sandy, Judy & Holley, Louie & Elizabeth, Dale, Johnny, Lucinda, Mark, Rebekkah, Sue, Mary and John, Janet E., Mary Ann, Jim Grainger

and especially to Muffin, Meurial, and Boo, who gave unconditional love.

Contributors

WARREN G. CLARK, RN, MS
Clinical Nurse Specialist, Psychiatry
Veterans Administration Medical Center
Johnson City, Tennessee
Adjunct Clinical Instructor
School of Nursing
East Tennessee State University

JEANNE DEVOS, RN, MA, MS
Associate Professor
School of Nursing
Marshall University
Huntington, West Virginia

THEODORE B. FELDMANN, MD
Assistant Professor
Director of Medical Student Education
Department of Psychiatry and Behavioral Sciences
University of Louisville
Louisville, Kentucky

STEVEN L. GILES, PhD
Chief, Psychology Service
Veterans Administration Medical Center
Johnson City, Tennessee
Assistant Clinical Professor
Department of Psychiatry and Behavioral Sciences
Quillen-Dishner College of Medicine
East Tennessee State University

ELEANOR HAVEN, RN
Project Manager
Veterans Administration—Regional Medical Education Center
Birmingham, Alabama

JO ANNALEE IRVING, MS, ARNP, CS
Assistant Professor
College of Nursing
University of Florida
Gainesville, Florida

PRISCILLA F. LEAVITT, PhD
Psychotherapist—Private Practice
Center for Individual and Family Counseling
Parkersburg, West Virginia

GIOVANNA B. MORTON, RN, BSN, MSN
Associate Professor
School of Nursing
Marshall University
Huntington, West Virginia

VINCE PISCITELLO, MSW
Instructional Systems Specialist
Veterans Administration—Information Systems Center
Birmingham, Alabama

MARTHA JOSEPHINE SNIDER, RN, EdD
Associate Professor and Director of Senior Studies
College of Nursing
University of Florida
Gainesville, Florida

NANCY D. STEPHENS, RD, MS
Clinical Dietician
Veterans Administration Medical Center
Huntington, West Virginia

DOREEN WARD, RN, BSN
Staff Nurse, Post Anesthesia Care Unit
Veterans Administration Medical Center
Huntington, West Virginia

Foreword

Medical and surgical nurses today are well schooled in acute care, having a solid foundation in and understanding of anatomy, physiology, pharmacology, and pathology. They are comfortable in the high-tech environment of ICUs, CAT scans, MRIs, organ transplantation, and joint replacements. However, patients with associated psychosocial problems or mental illnesses are often a source of confusion and misunderstanding. The nurse understands that these patients' needs may interfere with or even complicate an otherwise uncomplicated illness but she frequently requires help to recognize and respond to them appropriately.

Modern hospitals often provide, or have readily available, a wide variety of ancillary services, such as pastoral counselors, social workers, occupational therapists, behavioral scientists, and psychologists. Many institutions provide both inpatient and outpatient psychiatric services, and patients are often transferred to and from the medical and surgical services as conditions and symptoms warrant. Psychiatric backup is often available as needed. Yet it is the nurse, uniquely and absolutely essential for the 24-hour care and monitoring of patients, who must respond appropriately and accurately to the individuals under her care. For the medical-surgical nurse confronting someone with behavioral abnormalities, addiction, depression, psychiatric problems, or other forms of mental illness, what she does and how she does it often dictate the success of recovery.

Traditional psychiatric and psychiatric nursing texts are often written in mind-numbing, confusing jargon. The authors of this book have gone to great length, however, to filter and crystallize the basics of psychiatric and psychosocial illness into an easy to understand and easy to follow format. They have distilled the essence of a wide variety of mental illness, behavioral abnormalities, and even spiritual problems so that the nurse otherwise unfamiliar with these areas can utilize the information on a day-to-day basis and refer back to it again and again. Clinical manifestations of each condition are presented in outline form, and the assessment, planning, and intervention necessary for good nursing management are suitable for inclusion directly in the nursing care plans.

As a physician and surgeon in active practice, I have found that a patient's sense of health and well-being are often a very important factor in his recovery from illness. Over the years, the nurses I have most respected and learned from have recognized that they treat individuals, not just illnesses, and that successful intervention often depends as much on the alleviation of mental and emotional suffering as it does on the relief of physical suffering. This book provides the nurse with the skills and knowledge necessary to provide that relief, and I wholeheartedly recommend it for all those who care for the ill.

> The mind is its own place, and in itself,
> can make a Heaven of Hell, and a Hell of Heaven.
>
> John Milton, *Paradise Lost*
> Book I, 1667

Kenneth R. Hauswald, M.D., F.A.C.S.
Surgical Associates of Ashland
Ashland, Kentucky

Preface

> The trained nurse has become one of the great blessings of humanity, taking a place beside the physician and the priest, and not inferior to either in her mission.
>
> Sir William Osler

As nursing increases in complexity it becomes ever more crucial to recognize that the mind and body are, indeed, inseparable. This book uniquely addresses this dynamic interplay by combining classic concepts in psychiatric nursing and practical applications gained through personal experiences.

The primary theme of this book is that nurses care for patients with problems—*not* problem patients. This is particularly noteworthy when dealing with patients with psychiatric problems, since at those times respect for the individual assumes paramount importance. One characteristic of being human is to fear those things we do not understand. Often the nonpsychiatric nurse finds that she is fearful or uncomfortable caring for the medical-surgical patient who also has a psychiatric problem.

The basic tenet of this book is that skills in psychiatric nursing can be learned by any nurse and are applicable to any patient in the provision of holistic care. Each topic is presented in an easy-to-use, step-by-step format by authors with expertise in their respective subjects. Each of the book's 21 chapters is designed to stand alone and contains both basic and comprehensive information, including state-of-the-art knowledge not readily found in other resources. While writing style reflects each author's individuality, the organization of each chapter remains constant throughout the book. Although we are well aware that patients and health care providers can be of either sex, for convenience the patient will be referred to as "he," the nurse as "she," and the physician as "he," unless otherwise specified.

This book is designed to serve as a primary handbook on psychosocial intervention for medical-surgical and psychiatric nurses, nurse clinicians, nurse administrators, nurse researchers, and nurse educators as well as a reference book for nursing students. A broad spectrum of nurses in both inpatient and outpatient settings—hospital nursing units, community and home health organizations, nursing homes, hospices, mental health clinics, and agencies concerned with rehabilitation—will find the material essential to their practice. Allied health professionals who work closely with nurses—including physicians, social workers, psychologists, physical therapists, occupational therapists, and hospital chaplains—will discover enriching possibilities for their professions as well.

As Ernest Hemingway once said, "Life breaks everyone, and afterward many are strong in the broken places." This book presents many periods of brokenness that may be experienced throughout life. It is our philosophy that the unique mission of nursing is to render strength in those broken places.

THE EDITORS

Acknowledgments

This text was prepared with the assistance of many people. Special appreciation is given to the following people:

Alexander Nies
Mildred Mitchell-Bateman
Larry Smith
Henry Gernhardt
Ken Hauswald
Dorothea S. Strother

Contents

SECTION THREE

Addictive Behaviors and Chemical Dependency

SECTION FOUR

Special Concerns

SECTION FIVE
Other Issues

Appendices

The Greatest of These Is Love

Though I articulate the contemporary jargon of nursing,
If I have not understanding that touches the heartbeat of my patients,
I only generate chatter.

Though I boast of diplomas, awards and publications, and my skills reflect
the wonderment of technology,
If I have not mastered the gift of compassion,
My endeavors are hollow.

Though I impress my colleagues with my intellectual prowess and lofty
idealism,
If I offer not the instrument of self,
I serve my patients with mere activity.

Though I devote my very life to the profession of nursing and forfeit
personal desires,
If I become cynical, detached and fatigued to the point of indifference,
My energy is expended in futility.

Though I integrate the art and science of nursing, translate research into
clinical practice, and achieve professional notoriety,
If I do not notice wounded hearts and broken dreams,
My mission is not fulfilled.

I may be competent, dependable, and efficient,
But if I fail to communicate the language of love,
I practice nursing in vain.

Faith, hope, and love—these are all cravings of the human spirit . . . but
the greatest of these is love.

SECTION ONE

PSYCHIATRIC DISORDERS

Chapter 1

The Patient with Depression

Susan Lewis *Ruth Dailey Knowles Grainger*

I. STATEMENT OF PURPOSE

Depression is among the most common of psychiatric illnesses. It can be manifested as a primary disorder or a component of other psychiatric disorders such as bipolar disorder, substance abuse, schizophrenia, and personality disorders. Because individuals with the above manifestations may be hospitalized for physical conditions, it is important for the professional to know how to treat the depressed patient effectively. The purpose of this chapter is to provide the busy health care professional with some up-to-date approaches and interventions in order to deal more successfully with the hospitalized patient who is also depressed. Since depression is an almost expected part of physical illness, relief of some of the distressing feelings and associated symptoms can lower anxiety and speed the healing process.

II. OVERVIEW OF DEPRESSION

Depressed feelings occur so frequently in physically ill individuals that it has been said that depression is the most common of all psychiatric conditions for the hospitalized patient. This alteration in mood may range from a mild sadness to overwhelming despair. Depression is characterized by a feeling of sadness, emptiness, dissatisfaction, lowered self-esteem, inactivity, and self-deprecation. Clinical depression—depression requiring treatment, regardless of the etiology or the intensity of the symptomatology—will be the focus of this chapter.

A. Description of the Illness

Depression as a major health problem can occur at any point

in the life cycle, from the infant who fails to thrive (Frederickson, 1983), to the adult facing midlife, to the elderly person who contemplates suicide. Depression has been described as the expression of one's reaction to perceived loss and is a lowering of mood ranging in severity from the "Monday morning blues," to sadness, grief, or mourning, to immobilizing psychotic depression. Because it can be brought on by either hormonal/chemical changes or reactions to significant life changes, it can be anticipated, to some degree, to accompany all physical illnesses.

A depressed mood is not necessarily pathological. Depressed moods and feelings of sadness may be appropriate responses to loss. If the depression is profound enough to seriously interfere with the individual's overall functioning, and severe physical symptoms persist longer than two weeks, then the depression is said to be pathological.

Theories of the cause of depression are varied. Psychological theories focus on internalized anger and reaction to loss of significant objects or others. Because the related anger is unacceptable to the "self," it is turned inward, being automatically converted to guilt and depression. Another theory proposes that depression is related to biochemical abnormalities in the neurotransmitters at the synapses in the brain. Antidepressant medications are thought to work at the receptor sites in the synapses to increase the uptake of such chemicals as serotonin, norepinephrine, and dopamine.

In many cases of major depression, a precipitating factor can be identified with careful history, and the disorder may present with a clearly defined point of onset. In dysthymic disorders, symptoms may persist for a long period of time, and onset seems gradual and unclear. Depression may accompany the immobilization and apprehension experienced when the individual is hospitalized primarily for physical illness.

Depression may also be caused by or exacerbated through the side effects of medications. These include (Kaplan & Sadock 1985):

1. Antibacterials
2. Antihypertensives—most frequently reserpine, which is a MAO-depleting agent, but also hydralazine, clonidine, and guanethidine
3. Antineoplastics—mitotane, asparaginase
4. Antiparkinsonian drugs—levodopa, amantadine
5. Beta-adrenergic blockers—propranolol
6. Corticosteroids
7. Hormonal agents—estrogen, progesterone
8. Psychotropic drugs—antipsychotics, sedative-hypnotics, benzodiazepines, and narcotic analgesics

Depression can be related to a number of medical disorders, including (Kaplan & Sadock 1985):

1. Addison's or Cushing's disease
2. Cardiovascular disease
3. Gastrointestinal disorders
4. Hyperthyroidism/hypothyroidism
5. Infectious diseases—viral diseases such as mononucleosis
6. Malnutrition—especially protein and vitamin B deficiencies
7. Neoplastic disease—over 40% of cancer patients, especially those receiving chemotherapy, show symptoms of severe depression
8. Neurological conditions—brain tumors, Huntington's disease, neurofibromatosis, multiple sclerosis
9. Pancreatic disease
10. Rheumatoid arthritis—40–50% of these patients have depression

Depression is one phase of "bipolar disorder" (formerly called manic-depressive disorder), in which the depressed mood alternates with periods of elation and hyperactivity. (See also Chapter 3, "The Patient with Hyperactive or Manic Behavior.") Although much information is known about depression, knowledge of biochemical and psychological etiologies and specific mechanisms of action of treatment remain unclear.

B. Incidence

In the general population, depression is seen in 8–12% of males and in 20–26% of females (Weissman et al. 1987); however, some level of depression is seen in up to 85% of physically ill individuals.

There are a number of risk factors that increase the potential for depression (Weissman et al. 1987):

1. Sex—Approximately twice as many women as men are depressed.
2. Age—Depression may occur very early in childhood, but depression in both sexes peaks in the age group of 20–40 years.
3. Menopause—Although women 35–40 years of age have a high incidence of depression, studies show that there is no tendency for increased incidence during menopause.
4. Social class—There is no unique distribution pattern across socioeconomic classes.
5. Race—Recent data suggest that rates of major depression are lower among blacks.
6. Marital status—Highest rates of depression are found in separated or divorced persons.

7. Family history—Family studies show a 1.5- to 3-fold greater risk of depression among families with a history of depression.
8. Childhood experiences—There is evidence that disruptive, hostile experiences and a generally negative home life are risk factors for depression.
9. Personality traits—Studies of depressed patients suggest the following personality traits:
   a. Inability to cope with stress and anger
   b. Insecurity
   c. Oversensitivity
   d. Social awkwardness
   e. Dependency
   f. Tendency to worry
   g. Self-reproach
   h. Obsessionality
10. Recent life events—An excess of negative life events is found in depressed patients prior to the onset of a depressive episode.
11. Absence of an intimate relationship—Women who lack a close one-to-one relationship with someone in whom they can trust and confide are four times more likely than men to suffer a depression in the event of severe stress.

C. Clinical Manifestations

Major Depression

The patient who suffers from depression is consumed with an oppressive feeling of sadness and hopelessness. Life looks desolate and the patient's focus of attention is turned inward. Emotional characteristics include distorted thinking, leading to the "cognitive triad of depression": hopelessness about the self, hopelessness about the world in general, and hopelessness about the future (Beck et al. 1979). Accident-proneness may exist. Unrealistic attention to negative details, suspiciousness and paranoia, pessimism, guilt, self-blaming, sense of worthlessness, isolation, and feelings of emptiness, dissatisfaction, inadequacy, and depersonalization may exist. As depression deepens—or after a very deep depression has started to resolve and the client is feeling better with diminished psychomotor retardation—suicide becomes a real and present danger.

Suicidal ideation, though it may lead to actual suicide, is a common thought process in depressed patients. In an assessment of more than 400 clinically depressed patients done by one of us (R.D.K.G.), only 4 indicated that they did not experience suicidal ideation.

Physical characteristics associated with depression include a sad expression, crying, bowed posture, constipation, "aches and pains," poor concentration, malaise, and anxiety. The patient may have either a diminution or an increase in appetite. Consequently, either weight loss or weight gain may be seen. Sleep disturbance is a frequent complaint. Usually this is seen as insomnia, with early morning awakening (terminal insomnia) or frequent waking through the night. Occasionally, hypersomnia is found.

The depressed individual tends to dress in drab, dreary colors and isolate himself from others. Grooming may be poor. He may be demanding and irritable, easily distracted, and preoccupied with his somatic complaints. Even the smallest task, such as using the telephone or ordering a meal, may seem monumental to the depressed patient. Symptoms are typically worse in the morning, with some relief occurring toward evening.

Altered psychomotor behavior is seen as either psychomotor retardation or agitation. Psychomotor retardation is demonstrated by slowed speech of a low and monotonous character, decreased amount of speech (poverty of speech), slowed motor activity, slowed thinking (poverty of thought), muteness, decreased energy level, fatigue, constipation, inability to concentrate, memory impairment, and difficulty making decisions. Psychomotor agitation is manifested in restlessness and inability to sit still; pacing; wringing of hands; rubbing or pulling of hair, skin, or clothing; pressured speech; and irritability, with outbursts of anger.

Women are more likely to complain of depression, whereas men may describe secondary depressive phenomena such as difficulties at work or with achieving goals. The elderly may report failure or disappointment with self or family, or may focus on somatic symptoms. In the elderly, symptoms of depression—such as disorientation, poor memory, and distractibility—may be suggestive of dementia, and clarification of diagnosis may be difficult.

In some cases, depression can be so severe that psychosis, with delusions of persecution and hallucinations, occurs.

Dysthymic Disorder

The term dysthymic disorder is used to describe a chronic disturbance of mood involving depressed feelings or loss of interest in usual activities. The symptoms are basically the same as for major depression; however, they are less severe and persist over a longer period of time. Dysthymic disorder is manifested by a depressed mood occurring almost every day and lasting most of the day. For adults, at least two years' duration of symptoms is necessary for this diagnosis. The difference between major depression and dysthmic disorder is primarily based on intensity and duration of symptoms.

III. NURSING MANAGEMENT

The nurse must be knowledgeable about medical management of depressed patients, but since she may be working in any setting, the use of nonmedical interventions must be understood and utilized as appropriate. The following are some of the more up-to-date interventions that have been useful in the management of the depressed patient.

A. Assessment

1. Assess for the presence or absence of these symptoms:
   a. Depressed mood
   b. Sad affect
   c. Tearfulness
   d. Feelings of helplessness, hopelessness, and worthlessness
   e. Loss of interest in things previously enjoyed
   f. Change in appetite—increase or decrease
   g. Weight change—loss or gain
   h. Sleep disturbance—insomnia (especially early morning awakening) or hypersomnia
   i. Negative interpretation of events
   j. Memory problems
   k. Inability to concentrate or make decisions
   l. Decreased energy, with marked fatigue
   m. Decreased interest in sex
   n. Withdrawal and isolation of self from others
   o. Change in speech patterns—pressured or slowed speech
   p. Poverty of thought
   q. Poverty of speech
   r. Anxiety
   s. Suspiciousness and paranoia
   t. Self-blaming and feelings of inadequacy
   u. Preoccupation with inward-focused thoughts
   v. Irritability with and intolerance of others
   w. Distortion in thinking and judgment
2. Assess biological functioning—nutrition, elimination, and so on.
3. Assess for recent losses or other precipitating factors.
4. Assess available support systems and resources that might be appropriately used to ameliorate the depression.
5. Question for presence of suicidal or homicidal ideation and history of any past attempts.
6. Assess the degree of anger and irritability the patient is able to express.

7. Assess the presence of psychotic ideation—hallucinations or delusions (knowing that in all depression, there is a distortion in judgment).
8. Note physical appearance, grooming, manner of dress, mannerisms, and gait.
9. Question for alcohol or drug use, since this may contribute to depression or precipitate impulsive behavior.
10. Note presence of mood swings, with depression alternating with periods of elation or normalcy. This may indicate cyclothymic or bipolar disorder.
11. Question for history of repeated accidents or injuries.
12. Note self-blaming, self-accusation, and guilt.
13. Observe for alterations in psychomotor behavior—retardation or agitation.

B. Planning

Planning for nursing care of the depressed patient gives consideration to both physical and emotional needs. Careful observation and frequent reassessment of the patient's condition can alert the nurse to the potential for suicide.

C. Intervention

1. Prevention

   Prevention of depression involves teaching skills to help the patient gain more control over his emotions as well as his life. Specifically, the patient needs to learn to cope more appropriately with anger and loss.

   a. Help the patient to identify events that produce anger and recognize anger that may have been turned inward on the self.
   b. Teach skills to cope with anger effectively rather than "bottling it up inside."
   c. Teach techniques to assist the patient to deal with stress more effectively—progressive relaxation, positive visual imagery, autogenic self-talk.
   d. Encourage physical exercise such as walking or other motor activities.
   e. Encourage activities that increase self-esteem and promote a realistic and positive self-concept.
2. Treatment

   a. Hospitalization

      Depression may be so pronounced that psychiatric hospitalization is necessary. Hospitalization is frequently ordered when the patient is assessed to be dangerous to himself or others. The goals of hospitalization are to protect the patient from self-harm and to help him express anger and aggression in a constructive manner rather than turning it inward.

b. Electroconvulsive therapy (ECT)

Electroconvulsive therapy (ECT) may be used after the patient has been transferred to a psychiatric facility. ECT sometimes produces dramatic results in the treatment of depression; however, the patient must be carefully screened and selected for this type of treatment by his physician (Lewis et al. 1986). The possibility of ECT is often frightening to the patient and his family. The patient and family should be allowed to express their concerns about ECT and misconceptions should be clarified. The patient is required to sign a consent form indicating that he has been informed about the procedure and any risks involved and that he is agreeable to the treatment.

ECT is a treatment in which a grand mal seizure is induced by electric current to the frontal lobes. The patient is given an anesthetic and a muscle relaxant prior to treatment. Electrodes may be placed bilaterally; however, some practitioners believe that unilateral placement on the nondominant side produces less confusion. The number of treatments may vary according to the severity of the presenting problem and the patient's response to treatment.

Following ECT the patient may feel drowsy and confused, have a headache, and possibly experience some memory loss of the period of time just prior to the treatment. It is important for the nurse to be aware that the patient may feel extremely lost, lonely, and frightened following ECT. The nurse should be supportive, let the patient know she is checking on him frequently, and provide reorientation to the unit, other patients, and staff as necessary.

c. Outpatient treatment

Many patients who suffer from depression can be treated on an outpatient basis with a combination of psychotherapy and medication. Most cases of depression are time-limited, and the patient will improve with or without treatment; however, treatment certainly facilitates improvement and may prevent self-harm.

3. Medications

When depression is severe or has persisted for an extended period of time, antidepressant medications such as tricyclics or monoamine oxidase (MAO) inhibitors may be prescribed.

These medications can be highly effective in treating depression and are an important adjunct to psychotherapy.

a. Tricyclics

Tricyclic antidepressants are an important group of drugs and include amitriptyline, desipramine, doxepin, imipramine, nortriptyline, protriptyline, and others (see also Chapter 20, "Psychotropic Medications").

Although these drugs act on the central nervous system (CNS), their mechanism of action has not been completely elucidated. They are thought to cause an increase in the levels of neurotransmitters such as norepinephrine and serotonin at the synapse. Therapeutic response generally takes from two to three weeks; therefore, the patient should be made aware that he needs to continue the medication for a period of time long enough for an adequate trial.

Due to their anticholinergic properties, tricyclics may help the patient sleep, providing initial relief from insomnia, a frequent side effect of depression. The patient may experience side effects such as dry mouth, blurred vision, urinary retention, orthostatic hypotension, tachycardia, constipation, dizziness, and drowsiness. Low to moderate doses are initially administered to the patient, with dosages gradually increasing over a period of a few weeks to achieve greater therapeutic effect (Lewis et al. 1986).

b. MAO inhibitors

Monoamine oxidase (MAO) inhibitors have a relatively high toxicity and are often used when tricyclic antidepressants have proven ineffective. The exact mode of action is unknown, but it is thought that they directly increase the concentration of neurotransmitters by inhibiting MAO, an enzyme that breaks down norepinephrine.

The most common side effect seen with the use of MAO inhibitors is postural hypotension. Other potential side effects include lightheadedness, dizziness, anorexia, and insomnia. Careful monitoring of pulse rate and blood pressure is required.

MAO inhibitors can interfere with detoxification of certain chemicals and drugs by the liver. Despite the fact that it has always been advised that they should not be given in combination with tricyclics, MAO inhibitors and tricyclics are now being used together in select cases. Side effects appear to be no worse than when these drugs are used separately. If the drugs are given together, it is recommended that the MAO inhibitor be started *after* the tricyclic. The patient should be cautioned to avoid using medications containing ephedrine and over-the-counter preparations for colds, hay fever, or weight reduction, since the MAO inhibitors potentiate epinephrine and the combination may cause a severe hypertensive reaction (Taylor 1986).

Use of MAO inhibitors requires stringent dietary restriction, with abstinence from food containing tyramine or tryptophan. The patient on an MAO inhibitor cannot metabolize tyramine, and ingesting foods containing tyramine can precipitate a hypertensive crisis. Foods to be avoided include avocados; bananas; beer; broad beans; coffee (caffeine); cheeses such as cheddar, brie, camembert, and Stilton; Chianti wine; chicken livers; chocolate; cola; cream; figs; licorice; liver; meat tenderizer; pickled or kippered herring; raisins; sauerkraut; sherry wine; smoked salmon; snails; soy sauce; tea; yeast extract; and yogurt. Although the danger of hypertensive reactions remains a serious side effect, the actual occurrence is rare when caution is taken with diet and medication.

4. Nursing Actions
   a. Observe the patient closely at all times.
   b. Assess frequently for the presence of suicidal and/or homicidal ideation. Be aware that suicidal potential often increases as the patient becomes less depressed.
   c. Protect patient against self-harm or harm to others (see also Chapter 12, "The Patient with Suicidal Ideation").
   d. Use short, declarative sentences when talking with the severely depressed patient. His ability to remember and concentrate is diminished.
   e. Avoid phony cheerfulness with the patient. He may misinterpret this as insensitivity or lack of caring.
   f. Include the patient in unit activities even if his participation is limited. Depressed patients need to be with others and to feel accepted. Assign tasks that also extend the person outside himself, for example, writing to or calling family members, making objects for friends, or delivering cards or flowers to other individuals on the unit.
   g. Demonstrate respect for the patient.
   h. Listen with sensitivity when the patient speaks about his problems or feelings.
   i. Show interest and caring by spending time and talking with the patient.
   j. Monitor physical needs (nourishment, elimination, rest, and skin condition).

k. Allow the patient to make simple decisions such as what to eat or wear. Encourage him to delay making major decisions until his depression lifts, since he may make detrimental choices during the depths of depression. During depression, thinking is automatically distorted.

l. Maintain a consistent approach to the patient to create a sense of security.

m. Be sure that your communication to the depressed patient is honest, straightforward, and clear. It is quite acceptable to show honest concern for the patient, without reinforcing negative ideation and the depression.

n. Assign therapeutic tasks at which the patient can succeed, for example, doing something to help others, preparing something useful for the unit, and so on.

   A sense of accomplishment frequently lessens depression. Assign diversionary activities within the patient's capabilities to decrease self-centeredness and brooding. Try to schedule activities that can be completed within a relatively short period of time, for example, an occupational therapy session that can be completed between medications, before visiting hours, or after dinner. Encourage a progression of activities from the passive or sedentary to the more active and strenuous.

o. Encourage interaction with others. Even though the patient might not respond at first, he needs to be talked with, called by name, and listened to. Other patients may avoid the depressed patient, so the nurse may have to use ingenuity to increase contact with depressed patients.

p. Allow patient to finish his sentences, even though he may be speaking very slowly. Avoid finishing sentences for him. Respect the patient's need to communicate, even though it may be slowed by psychomotor retardation.

q. Avoid cheerfulness and reassurances that primarily reassure the nurse, not the patient. Superficial reassurances may be countertherapeutic.

r. Since some paranoia may exist, explain treatments and procedures fully, giving the patient any choices that may seem feasible. Advise the patient appropriately regarding medication. Know that the tendency toward negative ideation may encourage the patient to dwell on the potential negative aspects of medication.

s. Encourage exercise if at all possible. Strenuous activity helps reduce tension, provides a release of the energy that is attached to the anger (thereby reducing anger, hence depression), allows the best available antidepressant medication—the endorphins—to be created naturally in the brain. Exercise also helps combat constipation and promotes increased muscle tone and a sense of accomplishment and well-being.

t. Teach patient about the illness of depression—particularly that it is self-limiting. Emphasize that distorted thinking is characteristic of depression and that one is wisest not to trust one's perceptions at that time, because they are almost always negative.
u. Encourage any appropriate expression of anger, displeasure, or grief. In unchangeable situations the patient might punch a pillow, try shadowboxing, or use upper-body striking movements to help dissipate anger.
v. Teach problem-solving skills by asking the patient to list alternative actions, consider the rationale of each action, and evaluate which action might be in the patient's long-term best interest.
w. Teach antianxiety interventions if appropriate:
   - Progressive relaxation.
   - Breathing techniques to diminish anxiety
x. Teach thought-control techniques:
   - Replacement of negative, destructive self-statements with more accurate and realistic statements.
   - Dispute negative thoughts that are not useful (e.g., changing "I'm always going to feel this way" to "This will be over soon and I will survive").
   - Imagery to past events that were nondepressive, such as a time when the patient felt self-assured, loved, or successful. When the patient can image these, ask him to project them into the future to imagine when he will be experiencing these healthful emotions again.
   - Suggest that patients refrain from endlessly discussing their depression and symptomatology with family and friends, since this tends to internally reinforce the depression by focusing attention on it. It also may impair relationships with significant others because they tire of the depressive ideation or may be frightened or overwhelmed by the patient's symptomatology.
y. Teach behavioral management techniques:
   - Practice nondepressive behaviors even though the patient may not WANT to do them. That which was once enjoyable, when practiced, has a way of once again bringing some feelings of satisfaction even though depression may exist.
   - Encourage the patient to act "as if" things were different.

D. Evaluation/Expected Outcomes

Nursing care and patient progress can be evaluated through observable behaviors.

1. The nurse will:
   a. Protect the patient against self-harm or harm of others.
   b. Meet the physical needs until the patient can do this for himself.
   c. Provide an environment that the patient will view as accepting, consistent, secure, and nonthreatening.
2. The patient will:
   a. Understand depression as an illness, how it is precipitated, and what the patient can do to either prevent it or treat it if and when it appears.
   b. Increase his appropriate use of his support network.
   c. Increase his coping and decision-making skills and control over his own life.
   d. Learn to express feelings of guilt, self-loathing, anger, or worry in appropriate ways (e.g., stating the feelings in words rather than through physical symptoms or depression).
   e. Report delusions, hallucinations, and suicidal or homicidal ideation.
   f. Interact appropriately and realistically with staff, other patients, family, and friends.
   g. Identify stressors or situations that have in the past precipitated or contributed to depression, with a plan of action of how to either reduce, eliminate, or restructure his perception of the identified stressors or situations.
   h. Take medications as ordered.
   i. Increase attention to the environment and to others while decreasing introspection and self-centeredness.
   j. Participate in appropriate activities of the unit, family, or community.
   k. Continue in psychotherapeutic treatment.
   l. Identify, verbalize, and learn to utilize his personal strengths.

E. Evaluation for Referral

Patients with physical illnesses who are depressed may need referral to appropriate psychiatric practitioners for evaluation, consideration for medication, and treatment, since depression can hinder recovery.

IV. POTENTIAL OR ACTUAL NURSING DIAGNOSES

1. Communication, impaired verbal, related to
   - low self-esteem
   - slowed thought processes
   - decreased concentration
2. Coping, ineffective individual, related to
   - disturbances in mood
   - feelings of worthlessness and hopelessness
3. Decision making, impaired/ineffective, related to
   - anxiety
   - decreased concentration
   - disordered thought processes
   - low self-esteem
4. Grieving, dysfunctional, related to
   - perceived losses
   - feelings of guilt
   - internalized anger
5. Injury, potential for, related to
   - decreased attention to environment (see Violence, self-directed)
6. Powerlessness, related to
   - low self-esteem
   - feelings of worthlessness and hopelessness
7. Self-concept, disturbance in, related to
   - low self-esteem
   - feelings of guilt
   - delusions
   - feelings of worthlessness
8. Social isolation, related to
   - low self-esteem
   - delusions
   - low energy level
9. Thought process, altered, related to
   - impaired judgment
   - delusions
   - hallucinations
   - inability to make decisions
10. Violence, potential for, self-directed (suicidal), related to
    - suicidal ideation
    - feelings of guilt
    - internalized anger
    - feelings of hopelessness

11. Violence, potential for, other-directed (homicidal), related to
    - anger and/or hostility
    - delusions

V. SUMMARY

Patients with depression suffer tremendously, since for some reason, their perception of reality is distorted, negative self-statements and self-reproach abound, and these patients often appear to be desolate and temporarily unreachable. With wise and skillful nursing care, both physical and emotional, the patient will learn that depression is a temporary condition that can not only be treated, but can also be prevented.

References

American Psychiatric Association (1987). *Diagnostic and statistic manual of mental disorders* (3rd ed.-rev.). Washington, DC: APA.

Beck, A., Rush, A. J., Shaw, B. F., et al. (1979). *Cognitive therapy of depression.* New York: Guilford Press.

Clune, P. A., and Payne, D. B. (1982). *Psychiatric mental health nursing* (3rd ed.). New York: Medical Examination Publishing Co., Inc.

Frederickson, K. C. (1983). Depression—Specific behaviors and nursing interventions. In C. G. Adams and A. Macione (Eds.), *Handbook of psychiatric mental health nursing.* New York: John Wiley & Sons.

Kaplan, H. I., and Sadock, B. J. (1985). *Comprehensive textbook of psychiatry/IV.* Baltimore: Williams & Wilkins.

Knowles, R. D. (1984). Anxiety and the affective disorders. In J. Howe et al. (Eds.), *The handbook of nursing.* New York: John Wiley & Sons.

Knowles, R. D. (1984). *A guide to self-management strategies for nurses.* New York: Springer Publishing.

Lewis, S., McDowell, W. A., and Gregory, R. J. (1986). Saving the suicidal patient from himself. *RN Magazine*, Dec. pp. 26–28.

Rush, J. (1983). *Beating depression.* New York: Facts on File Publications.

Sacks, M. H. (1987). Depressive neurosis. In R. Michaels et al. (Eds.), *Psychiatry* (rev. ed.). New York: Lippincott.

Taylor, C. M. (1986). *Mereness' essentials of psychiatric nursing* (12th ed.). St. Louis: C. V. Mosby Co.

Veterans Administration (April 28, 1982). *Program Guide—Nursing Service* (G-10, M-2, Part V). Washington, DC: U.S. Government Printing Office.

Weissman, M. M., Merikangas, K., and Boyd, J. H. (1987). Epidemiology of affective disorders. In R. Michaels et al. (Eds.), *Psychiatry* (rev. ed.). New York: Lippincott.

Chapter 2

The Patient with Anxiety

Ruth Dailey Knowles Grainger

I. STATEMENT OF PURPOSE

This chapter is designed to provide specific information for the staff nurse on a general hospital unit who is dealing with patients exhibiting anxiety-related behavior. This chapter is less of a discussion of the "why's" of patients' anxieties than an explanation of the effective interventions the nurse can use when faced with patients who are anxious.

II. OVERVIEW OF ANXIETY

A. Description of the Illness

Anxiety is a feeling of apprehension manifested by feelings of impending doom, dread, and uneasiness that is evoked by some perceived threat to the individual. Mild to moderate anxiety helps an individual to focus attention on immediate details and may even enhance the ability to deal with anxiety-producing behavior. On the other hand, high anxiety narrows perceptions, decreases the level of functioning, and may lead to inappropriate behavior, illness or somatic complaints, and immobilization or panic.

The nurse must remember that the function of anxiety in the patient is to set protective defenses into motion and to make that individual feel more secure. Unfortunately, many manifestations of anxiety work to the contrary by actually diminishing security feelings in the patient.

The nurse can serve in a highly useful role, since she:

1. Understands that the anxiety is a protective move.
2. Accepts the expression of anxiety.
3. Helps patient to understand it better.

4. Teaches coping strategies to use now and in the future.

B. Incidence

Since some degree of anxiety accompanies all systemic dysfunction, it is to be expected in all hospitalizations and is experienced in varying degrees in each ill or injured individual. However, high levels of anxiety and stress interfere with functioning and healing, so the nurse needs specific interventions to counteract the potential negative effects of these emotions.

C. Clinical Manifestations

Clinical manifestations include tachycardia, hyperventilation, anorexia, vertigo, pallor, chest pain, respiratory distress, dry mouth, dilated pupils, itching/hives, flushing, nausea, tremors, insomnia, dysphagia, sighing, diarrhea, weakness, sweating, and cramps.

III. NURSING MANAGEMENT

A. Assessment

On the hospital unit, anxiety is frequently manifested in several ways, from the useful mild level of increased alertness, with perhaps more questions than usual, to extremely anxious behaviors of crying, pacing, hand wringing, and even panic attacks.

Assessment questions the nurse might seek to answer from either the chart, patient, or visitors include:

1. What are the medical diagnoses?
2. What are the nursing diagnoses?
3. What are the relationships between the two?
4. What does the patient think is causing the anxiety?
5. What happens immediately before the anxiety attack?
6. How often have the symptoms occurred before?
7. What did the patient do to treat or help alleviate the symptoms in the past?
8. Is there a relationship between anxiety and:
   a. Diet (e.g., high sugar concentrations cause anxiety in some patients).
   b. Activity level and exercise (e.g., some people become "positively addicted" to physical activity, such as running and tennis, as an intervention for anxiety and depression).
   c. Medical problems (e.g., irritability and anxiety that may be present in strokes, brain tumors, and so on).

d. Alterations in living habits (e.g., first time in years to sleep alone).
e. Side effects/toxic effects of medications (euphoria or anxiety may be present when patient is taking corticosteroids and others).
f. Side effects of withdrawal from addictive substances:
   - Smoking (inability to have cigarettes can cause intense craving and anxiety from the deprivation).
   - Alcoholic beverages (what appears to be anxiety may be some of the first signs of alcohol withdrawal).
   - Illicit drugs (anxiety can be caused by withdrawal symptoms).
   - Prescribed or over-the-counter drugs customarily taken at home.
   - Types of food eaten (e.g., if the person is accustomed to a "caffeine fix" every morning, inability to get coffee may cause anxiety and headaches; ingestion of chocolate can cause tachycardia and sleeplessness because of excessive theobromine, which acts like caffeine in the system).

9. What is happening in terms of recent life-change events within the family?
10. Are there family activities that need to be handled or information that needs to be shared/gathered to reduce the patient's level of anxiety?
11. Are there actual changes in the patient's mental status (e.g., confusion, irritability, depression, mental fatigue, feelings of loss of control, or fear of overdependency)?
12. What are the thoughts that are disturbing to the patient?
    a. To what degree are they rational?
    b. Is further factual information related to diagnosis, treatment, nursing interventions, or medications needed?
    c. Are thoughts primarily "worries"?
    d. Can their "usefulness" be discussed and explored?
13. To what degree is there a support system of close friends, family, and co-workers?
14. How can the support system be utilized to decrease the patient's anxiety?
15. What part of the anxiety reaction troubles the patient the most? (The skilled nurse can use this information in planning treatment and providing intervention when the patient becomes extremely anxious.)

B. Planning

Planning for the anxious patient should be based on a thorough nursing assessment taking into consideration the nature and intensity of the patient's symptoms.

C. Intervention

1. Prevention

   Because anxiety is an expected concomitant with all hospitalizations, prevention of initial anxiety is almost impossible. However, there are interventions that the nurse can use to decrease initial anxiety and help to prevent later high anxiety from occurring. As the nurse uses—and teaches the patient—the self-management strategies for controlling anxiety (listed under "Nursing actions"), the patient should become far more resourceful in preventing and/or minimizing high anxiety in the future.

2. Treatment

   Treatment of anxiety should be multimodal, ranging from the therapeutic use of the nurse's voice, to the nurse teaching the patient emergency anxiety-management breathing techniques, to long-term psychotherapy. The purpose of this section is to describe what the nurse can do to intervene in the anxiety of patients so that they are more functional, heal quicker, are better able to cooperate with treatment regimens, and learn, hopefully for a lifetime, how to manage their anxiety better. Since high anxiety interferes with the efficient working of the autoimmune system, the resulting stress has a way of exacerbating almost any physical condition; therefore, the reinterpretation (reframing) of stressful events can reduce anxiety and the resulting state of stress.

   Treatment of anxiety, however, requires knowledge, skill, empathetic warmth, and perserverance. Whereas the staff nurse may be able to provide many interventions, it is important that any nurse KNOW her own limitations and refer those patients needing more in-depth assistance to the nurse-psychotherapist, social worker, psychologist, or psychiatrist.

3. Medications

   Antianxiety (anxiolytic) medications can be utilized under medical management and are covered in detail in Chapter 20, "Psychotropic Medications."

4. Nursing Actions

   a. Let the patient know that you are aware of his anxiety and that you take it seriously. Listen respectfully to what the patient has to say.
   b. Be available to the patient, checking in with him often if this seems to ease anxiety. If patient is in a panicky state, stay with him until he is less panicked.

c. Maintain a calm manner, using short declarative sentences and utilizing a soft but firm voice (which can imply to the patient that you will provide the external controls needed).
d. If possible, move a highly anxious patient to a smaller physical environment to minimize external stimuli. Help the patient to verbalize anxiety and remind the patient, without using inappropriate reassurances, that the anxiety is time-limited, thus planting seeds of relief to come.
e. Initially, *present the familiar* to the patient by reflecting to the patient aspects of his behavior that are familiar (e.g., sitting in a posture similar to the patient's, pacing your movements to about the same rate as the patient's, listening well enough to hear highly valued words the patient says and using these in the discussion, and matching your voice tone and rate to the patient's).
f. Eventually make changes in your voice that make it:
   - Lower in pitch
   - Softer
   - Slower

   These changes in the nurse's voice are often contagious to the patient who listens, and the patient may begin to respond in like manner. A second reason for the nurse to speak lower, softer, and slower is the "biofeedback" message to the nurse that she is calm, whether this is factual or not. This is a major, immediate action that the nurse can take with most anxious patients.
g. The nurse helps her patient best when she encourages expression of thoughts and feelings about illness, dependency, and other concerns rather than inappropriately reassuring the patient when anxiety exists. If the patient's thoughts and feelings about events are not identified and expressed (preferably in an appropriate way), these stresses can continue to influence the behavior of the patient, many times in destructive or inappropriate ways (e.g., through restless anxiety, depression, acting out, or somatic complaints).
h. Allow full expression as appropriate; however, this should not take on the character of an endless recital, since that may be reinforcing to the anxiety.
i. Assist patient in identifying threats or stresses in his personal environment that might be removed.
j. Since perceptions are narrowed when anxiety is increased, realize that the patient may have difficulty making decisions, problem solving, attending, or remembering.

k. Teach the patient the effectiveness of altering negative self-statements to more realistic ones, to produce less unnecessary anxiety. Are the statements the patient is making to himself or others useful, true, productive, and in his best interest?

l. Teach the patient to monitor thoughts that are precursors of anxious feelings. Teach patient to question whether a thought is rational or irrational and, if irrational, how to dispute it with a rational thought. For example, the patient may be very anxious and saying, "I just *know* the lab tests are going to be positive and I will die if I have 'X' diagnosis!" The nurse might question the patient about the usefulness of determining, before the results are in, that the outcome is necessarily negative. She might have the patient dispute his own negative statement with, "What evidence do I have at this time for my assumption?" or "Won't it be a waste of all of my energy now if the results are negative?"

m. Teach patient to make positive self-statements. Have the patient make a list of positive self-statements to use when anxious, for example:
   - "I have been anxious before and I got over it."
   - "This feeling will leave me soon."
   - "Nothing actually happens to me when I get anxious; I am only uncomfortable."

n. Teach the patient to question the rationality of his anxiety, for example:
   - "What is the worst thing that can happen to me in this situation?"
   - "What is the probability of that occurrence?"
   - "What is the cosmic significance of this event?"

o. Teach the patient to rate his own anxiety level on a scale of "0–10" (0 = asleep, 10 = complete panic). Ask the patient to identify his current anxiety level, then engage in breathing or other stress-management techniques, and immediately assess his anxiety level afterwards. This is a way to convince the patient that he can successfully control his anxiety on his own.

p. Teach patient to attempt to lower anxiety at frequent intervals during the day in order to prevent the cumulative effect of anxiety in the evenings.

q. Teach the patient to use breathing and relaxation techniques for anxiety that is moderate (levels 4–6 on the anxiety scale).

- Take a deep breath, hold for a count of three, then let it out. Do this 1–3 times, then assess anxiety level afterwards.
- Quiet breathing technique. With each expiration, have the patient mentally say a repetitive word (e.g., one, calm, or peace). This gives the mind something to do OTHER THAN worry, while at the same time providing a distraction from the anxiety.
- Progressive relaxation is the relaxation of the entire body, starting at one body part and then progressing to the next body part until relaxation is complete. Start first with relaxing the toes, balls of feet, arches, and so on, moving up the body to the shoulders, down the arms, returning to the back of the neck, then bringing relaxation up over the scalp to flow down over the face, relaxing fully.

r. Teach the patient to do thought stopping. First, the patient identifies those thoughts that are troublesome to him. Second, he identifies several visual images that are very pleasant and rewarding to him. Third, every time he identifies the negative thought entering his awareness, he startles himself by either yelling "STOP IT," clapping his hands together, or (if in polite company) yelling in his mind. Fourth, he immediately flashes into his mind the pleasant thought, thinks about it for a second or so, and then goes on about the activities of his day. Use of this cognitive-behavioral technique will quickly diminish the frequency of the unwanted thought by failing to reinforce it by its presence.

s. Teach patient to use anxiety as a body signal that alerts him that there is a threat to the organism. Is the purpose of this anxiety one of protection, alerting the individual to something that needs to be done or that additional information is needed, or is it alerting the patient to survival issues?

t. Teach the patient to use "anchoring" to bring on a relaxed state:
   - Have the patient adopt a relaxed state (physically comfortable, perhaps remembering a very relaxing and tranquil experience). Teach the patient to bring up these memories or pleasant future anticipations that encourage the mind to become more relaxed.
   - When the patient is very relaxed, ask him to press his forefinger and thumb of the nondominant hand together at the time of the greatest relaxed feeling. This provides

the brain with a "kinesthetic (feeling) anchor" or association that will assist the patient in once again finding the relaxed scene and the relaxed feeling.

- When the patient needs this relaxed feeling in the future, he need only touch the forefinger and thumb together to "trigger" (recall) the return of the relaxed feeling associated with this special gesture.

u. Teach the patient to use imagery and affirmations, to imagine himself being successful in an anxiety-provoking situation.

- First, using the above anchoring gesture, have patient imagine the feared situation.
- Next, instead of worrying about the anxiety-provoking situation, have the patient "rewrite the script" so that the outcome is positive and successful.
- Ask the patient to carefully construct this successful scene, paying close attention to what he sees, says, feels, and does, and to what others say and do. This will vivify the scene and make it more persuasive to the unconscious mind.

v. Teach the patient anxiety interventions that include, if possible, exercise. (Breathing techniques described in entry "q" above work well on anxiety levels of approximately 1–6, but more physical interventions such as strenuous exercise or psychotropic medications are usually necessary for levels 7–10.)

w. Emphasize that regression is a defense mechanism often seen as a natural part of illness and that a certain amount of regressive behavior is useful in the healing process (e.g., staying in bed, temporarily setting aside employment responsibilities in order to heal the body, and accepting the amount of dependency that is necessary during hospitalization). Explaining this to the patient often relieves some unnecessary anxiety.

x. Sometimes, anxiety is caused by unrealistic hopes, standards, and expectations for self and others. The patient may be encouraged to examine these attitudes to determine if any changes in interpretation or expectation might help him to use different tactics or resources in order to get needs met.

y. Be available to the patient or tell him whom to contact during periods of high anxiety.

z. Realize that anxiety is a feeling of loss of control. Any nursing interventions that can help the patient gain actual control over aspects of the situation, himself, or his health, emotions, thoughts, and future will help to alleviate the anxiety and/or to employ it appropriately.

D. Evaluation/Expected Outcomes

The patient will be able to:

1. Report anxiety when present, using words.
2. Rate the level of anxiety (on a 0–10 scale) and report this level.
3. Determine the major predisposing circumstances or situations that seem to engender anxiety.
4. Identify anxiety-provoking situations and determine if they are:
   a. Signals to do something
   b. Messages that the body/mind needs protection
5. Identify usual thought patterns precipitating anxiety and determine if they are:
   a. Rational or irrational thoughts
   b. Worries or useful for problem solving
6. On his own, select and effectively utilize anxiety-management techniques.
7. Control "not-useful" thinking.
8. Control "not-useful" behaviors that produce anxiety.
9. Decrease somatic complaints.
10. Express hostility and anger appropriately.
11. Alter diet, exercise, living habits, or medications to reduce anxiety.
12. Realize that anxiety is a state of mind and can be controlled by altering the interpretation (or misinterpretation) of any event or situation.
13. Realize that anxiety is temporary and understandable, and will fluctuate during hospitalization.
14. Utilize support systems appropriately.
15. Exhibit useful and appropriate ways to get needs met.

E. Evaluation for Referral

All patients who exhibit anxiety do not need to be referred to a mental health professional for counseling. Anxiety, in the hospital, is usually related to procedures, diagnosis, separation from family, and response to environmental and personal stresses there. It would be appropriate for the nurse to seek referral of the patient, for psychological/psychiatric or medical services, if the patient:

1. Obsesses about a procedure or event to the degree that mental confusion and impaired judgment are evident.
2. Is having disruption of sleep for more than two nights.
3. Is so upset that he is unable to eat.

4. Has repeated bouts of crying, pacing, or other extreme anxiety behaviors.
5. Has more than one panic attack.
6. Reports clinical manifestations that either last for several hours or occur frequently, such as tachycardia, chest pain, respiratory distress, or excessive sweating.
7. Is excessively withdrawn.
8. Is overtly hostile to the health care professionals and refuses treatments.
9. Is experiencing severe life-changes or losses while hospitalized (e.g., a family member was killed or severely injured in this patient's accident).
10. Verbalizes suicidal ideation.
11. Does not respond to the nurse's use of all the techniques and interventions suggested in this chapter for the purpose of lowering anxiety.

IV. POTENTIAL NURSING DIAGNOSES

1. Anxiety, related to a perceived threat to any aspect of the self
2. Maladaptive coping patterns, related to
   - learned somatization as an unconscious defense against anxiety
   - internalization of anxiety, causing free-floating anxiety and/ or depression
3. Sleep-rest activity, disturbance in, related to
   - anticipation of inability to sleep
   - worry
   - anxious feelings
   - agitation

V. SUMMARY

The nurse is the health professional in one of the most influential positions with the anxious patient because she is with the patient for 24 hours a day. Through utilization of appropriate nursing actions, the skilled, understanding, and therapeutic nurse can not only affect the thoughts and feelings of the anxious patient, but also help prepare the patient for more control when anxiety is encountered in the future. This "quick reference" for the nurse dealing with the anxious patient on a nonpsychiatric hospital unit is based on the belief that nurses can know WHAT to do only when they know HOW to do it, because the desire to be helpful, the intent to be therapeutic, and the warmth to reach out to the anxious patient are already there.

References

Benson, H. (1975). *The relaxation response.* New York: Avon Books.

Discusses the physiological responses to stress, and the interrelationship between emotion and the effect of the relaxation response. Also included are relaxation exercises.

Brailler, L. (1982). *Successfully managing stress.* Los Altos, CA: National Nursing Review.

Up-to-date and comprehensive, this guide to the holistic treatment of stress by a leading nurse therapist is as useful for the professional as it is for the anxious patient.

Cousins, N. (1983). *The healing heart: Antidotes to panic and helplessness.* New York: W. W. Norton and Co.

Up-beat book for patients to read to gain more emotional control when combating physical illness.

Emery, G. (1982). *A new beginning: How you can change your life through cognitive therapy.* New York: Simon and Schuster.

Application of cognitive therapy to anxiety and depression, and a comprehensive overview of the field. Highly readable and practical.

Emery, G., and Campbell, J. (1986). *Rapid relief from emotional distress.* New York: Rawson Associates.

An excellent book to assign to patients in emotional distress.

Helmstetter, S. (1987). *The self-talk solution.* New York: William Morrow and Company.

Details procedures for talking appropriately to the self, using effective thought processes rather than destructive ones.

Knowles, R. D. (1981). Managing anxiety. *American Journal of Nursing, 81,* 110–111.

Deals with anxiety by awareness/leveling techniques and the use of breathing exercises. Includes the problem intervention, rationale, and evaluation of stress-management techniques.

Knowles, R. D. (1984). *A guide to self-management strategies for nurses.* New York: Springer Publishing.

Many practical interventions to help control one's environment, thoughts, behaviors, and feelings are presented in this book. The script of a relaxation, self-hypnosis tape the reader can make is included.

Knowles, R. D. (1984). Anxiety and the affective disorders. In J. Howe et al. (Eds.), *The handbook of nursing.* New York: John Wiley & Sons.

Overview and nursing interventions for the anxious patient, in outline form.

Siegel, B. S. (1986). *Love, medicine and miracles: Lessons learned about self-healing from a surgeon's experience with exceptional patients.* New York: Harper and Row Publishers.

Inspiring book about what the patient can do to help himself heal, keep his anxiety low, and be more in control of his life.

Chapter 3

The Patient with Hyperactive or Manic Behavior

Susan Lewis *William A. McDowell*
Robert J. Gregory

I. STATEMENT OF PURPOSE

When aware of the existence of manic behavior or hyperactivity in a patient, the nurse is often a key figure in patient management and intervention efforts. Problem behavior or crisis situations can often be avoided or minimized if the patient is handled in a therapeutic manner. This chapter gives the nurse an understanding of the dynamics involved and facilitates management of the patient's behavior.

II. OVERVIEW OF HYPERACTIVE OR MANIC BEHAVIOR

A. Description of the Illness

(*Note:* The term manic-depressive illness is now referred to as bipolar disorder. The terms may be used interchangeably, with the word "manic" being used to describe the hyperactive or elated phase of the illness. It is important to note that hyperactive behavior may be caused not only by bipolar disorder, but also by a number of other conditions.)

Some individuals defend against extreme feelings of anxiety, loneliness, inadequacy, and failure by means of excessive talkativeness, hyperactivity, and elated mood. Indeed, the elated mood may be so pronounced and sustained that the individual expresses the belief that every good thing is possible and every wish will be fulfilled. Ideas may emerge in a rapid, fluid-like fashion; thinking seems effortless and memory is sharp. The individual may show a quick but superficial wit and may exhibit a sense of self-security that masks and minimizes fears. The individual may be aggressive, opinionated, and ready to talk with conviction on any and every topic. The ego seems to be unrestrained, and ideas pour out so rapidly that the individual may express only segments of ideas. A conversation may quickly jump from topic to topic. With a speedy recognition of persons and objects, the individual is likely to be domineering, irritable, and hypercritical of anything that interferes with personal plans, and may exhibit excessive motor activity. When limits are imposed on behavior, the individual can become noisy, belligerent, and even violent. Insight is poor, for attention is focused on the environment rather than the self.

Such an individual usually has some reality orientation, but, as stated above, lacks insight and shows poor judgment. The hyperactive patient is often a poor candidate for clinic or day care center, since he exhibits disruptive behavior to cover or defend himself. The patient himself may not admit that anything is wrong.

Although behaving with arrogance, the manic patient actually feels worthless and useless. Feelings of worthlessness may lead to beliefs of not deserving to have needs met, which in turn leads to the perception of rejection by others. Only by manipulating others may the individual satisfy demands. This manipulation defends against failure and provides a false sense of power and control over those manipulated.

The manic patient's excessive demands prevent any one person from satisfying all of the patient's needs. As more people reject the demanding patient, however, anxiety increases, thereby increasing demands. Elation and hyperactivity are an appeal for love and a protection from depression. Use of amphetamines, or even caffeine, may initiate or aggravate the personality dynamics described.

B. Incidence

It is estimated by the American Psychiatric Association that 0.4%–1.2% of the adult population have bipolar disorder (DSM III, 1980). There is a significant hereditary component in bipolar disorder. The first manic episode usually occurs before age 30.

C. Clinical Manifestations

The hyperactive or manic patient manifests a number of characteristic behaviors, outlined below. While some of these characteristics appear contradictory, wide variations in behavior patterns do occur among these patients. Awareness of these behavioral characteristics will facilitate appropriate intervention.

1. Extreme hyperactivity

2. Aggressive, extroverted behavior
3. Boldness, overconfidence
4. Over-responsiveness to environmental stimuli, distractibility
5. Low frustration tolerance, short attention span
6. Hostility, emotional irritability, and destructive acting-out
7. Suspicion of others (paranoia)
8. Manipulative behavior, with attempts to intimidate staff or "pit" them against each other
9. Assumption of a supervisory role
10. Expansive ideas, delusions of grandeur, planning "big deals," flight of ideas
11. Constant, rapid, and/or loud talking with skipping or slurring of words
12. Use of profanity and obscene language
13. Extravagance and squandering of money
14. Use of garish combinations of clothing and jewelry
15. Decoration of surroundings with colorful cloths, pictures, or paintings
16. Frequent mood changes and fluctuations from euphoria to depression
17. Preoccupation with activities that preclude eating, eliminating, resting, or sleeping
18. Hypersexual behavior

III. NURSING MANAGEMENT

Short-term goals of nursing care are to provide a safe environment that promotes health and minimizes hyperactive behavior. Long-term goals are to promote stabilization of the patient's condition and normalization of behavior.

A. Assessment

1. Obtain a thorough psychosocial and health history.
2. Evaluate health status: nutrition, elimination, activity level, and sleep patterns. Exhaustion can occur after extended periods of hyperactivity.
3. Question for a family history of affective disorders, other mental illnesses, or alcoholism.
4. Note that hyperactivity and elated mood can be associated with certain organic conditions or chemical or hormonal imbalances: seizure disorder, neoplasm, infection, or hyperthyroidism.
5. Assess drug history. Hyperactivity can be a side effect of certain drugs including: steroids, levodopa, bromides, isoniazid, amphetamines, and caffeine.

6. Question for a history of cycling between elated and depressed moods.
7. Note present behavior patterns: increased motor activity, irritability, agitation, spending, or grandiose plans.
8. Assess environmental influences on behavior. Environmental stimuli can contribute to hyperactivity
9. Observe grooming and manner of dress.
10. Examine any relationships between hyperactive behavior and interpersonal contact with others including patients, staff, and visitors.

B. Planning

Planning of nursing care for the manic or hyperactive patient should be based on a comprehensive nursing assessment and subsequent nursing diagnosis. Modification of the nursing care plan should be based on frequently scheduled reassessments of the patient's status and evaluation of nursing care.

C. Intervention

1. Prevention

   Prevention of hyperactive or manic episodes is focused on stressing the importance of taking medication, especially lithium carbonate, as prescribed by the physician. Monitoring of serum lithium levels provides information on the therapeutic range of lithium in the patient's blood stream.

   It is also important for the nurse to observe the patient's behavior closely in order to be alert to early clues to changes in mood.

2. Treatment

   Treatment of the manic or hyperactive patient encompasses three goals. The first is to increase the patient's awareness of his illness and his sensitivity to changes in his symptoms so that intervention can begin early. Compliance with medication and the importance of living a structured life should be stressed. The second goal of treatment is to help the patient learn to cope with stress and disappointment. The third goal of treatment is to help the patient improve interpersonal relationships. Even between mood swings these patients have difficulty with interpersonal relationships, since they lack sensitivity to the feelings of others.

   One of the immediate objectives in handling the hyperactive or manic patient is to help the patient feel as accepted and as secure as possible. This will decrease anxiety and protect the patient from injury to self or others. In the long run, this will help maintain physical health. A consistent attitude of kind firmness is more helpful than either permissiveness or extreme rigidity.

External control can give the patient a greater sense of security, reduce anxiety, and help the patient feel that the nurse is concerned. Setting limits on behavior can also help prevent injury to the patient or to others.

All staff should be fully aware of any nursing care plan implemented and be careful to use a consistent approach. The hyperactive patient may learn what aggravates staff members and attempt to manipulate the staff or pit them against each other. The manner in which the patient is approached will often determine responses. The elated patient frequently argues and thus needs simple explanations that leave no room for argument. Criticism of the patient may only reinforce existing feelings of inadequacy.

Dehydration, weight loss, and malnutrition are characteristics of the hyperactive patient. The patient may be much too busy to worry about physical needs such as eating, sleeping, and eliminating. This type of patient also has a tendency to dress flamboyantly, garishly, and inappropriately, sometimes even running about in the nude.

The hyperactive patient has a very short attention span. The patient's interests may change so rapidly that a demand may be forgotten if it is postponed. The patient cannot be restricted in everything, so some demands must be met to limit others. Partial satisfaction of a demand may reduce a grandiose demand to a more manageable size, and, with guidance, the patient may be able to use excess energy productively in solitary activities.

Hyperactivity can be escalated by environmental stimuli. Therefore, it is best to have as calm and subdued an atmosphere as possible. Lightweight or small furniture can be used as weapons by the patient and should be removed from the room. Positive reinforcement may encourage appropriate behavior.

3. Medications

Attending physicians may prescribe psychotropic medication. Lithium carbonate is a naturally occurring element often used to control manic behavior, although the exact mode of action is not known. The safety margin between therapeutic levels is 0.5–1.5 meq/L, and the full beneficial effect is noted 6–10 days after initiation of therapy. To reduce the danger of lithium intoxication, sodium intake must remain at normal levels. Renal functioning should be within normal limits for patients receiving lithium.

Neuroleptics such as Navane, Haldol, Thorazine, Mellaril, Prolixin, and Stelazine may also be used to help control or subdue behavior, particularly on a short-term basis while therapeutic levels of lithium are being established. (See also Chapter 20, "Psychotropic Medications.")

4. Nursing Actions

The nine key actions outlined below can assist the nurse in managing the hyperactive or manic patient during hospitalization.

a. Set limits on patient's behavior:
   - Restrict the patient to the ward if disruptive to other areas.
   - Limit the patient's use of the telephone, especially hospital or business phones.
   - Call on hospital police to return the patient to the unit if necessary. (*Note:* The legality of limiting a patient's privileges may vary according to geographical area. In general, a *psychiatric* patient may be restricted to a closed unit or placed on voluntary admission status. This may apply differently in a medical-surgical area; however, a primary goal of care is to protect the patient from harm to self or others.)
   - Make the patient aware of limits as early as possible in the treatment period.
   - Provide one-to-one observation of the patient if it is necessary to calm him.
   - Medicate to calm the patient, if need be. Remain alert to behavior changes and medicate as needed.

b. Use a consistent approach with the patient:
   - Become familiar with the patient's moods and reactions to staff members.
   - Be alert to changes in behavior or an increase in irritability or activity level. Begin nursing intervention as soon as changes in behavior are noted.
   - Physical distance lessens the patient's misperception of an attack.

c. Listen respectfully and calmly without arguing and with little comment. Use neutral, matter-of-fact responses.
   - Use a firm, calm, low-pitched voice with a coaxing quality.
   - Avoid falling in with the patient's entertaining manner and playful behavior.
   - Recognize your own feelings. Do not show anger or scold the patient.
   - Avoid long conversations and explanations.

d. Monitor physical needs such as diet, elimination, rest, and exercise.
   - Provide food that the patient can eat "on the go."
   - Encourage intake of fluids.
   - Encourage rest.
   - Monitor elimination and take appropriate nursing actions.
   - Encourage appropriate dress.

e. Help the patient channel excess energy.
   - Encourage activities that can be completed in a short time such as: writing experiences, tearing rags for rugs, doing housekeeping chores, making paper maché, pounding copper, or helping the staff make beds. Ask the occupational therapist or volunteer services for crafts or activities that the patient can complete at the bedside, such as model building, doodle art, and so on.
   - Taking long walks on a regular basis may help the patient channel energy. Patient should be accompanied by a staff member or possibly a volunteer.
   - Facilitate and encourage any desire or interest of the patient to write or draw.

f. Use distractibility and suggestibility to deal with demands or offensive behavior.

g. Simplify the environment and decrease sensory stimulation.
   - Provide a private room as far away from other daily activities as possible. Other patients may become quite irritated by the manic patient.
   - Eliminate pictures and colorful drapes.
   - Remove unnecessary furniture.
   - Use subdued colors and patterns for walls.
   - Use lighting that is subdued.
   - Decrease the noise level in the environment.

h. Encourage any behavior approaching normalcy.

i. Provide education to the patient and family for early detection of symptoms and early intervention.

D. Evaluation/Expected Outcomes

1. The nurse will:
   a. Protect the patient from self-harm or harm to others.
   b. Modify the environment to provide safety and decrease stimuli.
   c. Place limits on the patient's inappropriate or destructive behavior.

d. Maintain consistency in the treatment plan.
e. Assign tasks to keep the patient occupied.
f. Avoid being manipulated by the patient's playful behavior and entertaining ways.

2. The patient will:
   a. Dress in an appropriate manner.
   b. Eat a nutritionally balanced diet.
   c. Adhere to ward routine and regulations.
   d. Find appropriate outlets for anger.
   e. Sleep for 5–7 hours/night.
   f. Complete assigned tasks.
   g. Take medication as prescribed.
   h. Remain oriented to reality.
   i. Gain an understanding of his condition and identify situations that may precipitate symptoms of either elated or depressed mood.
   j. Seek intervention when elation or depression begins.

E. Evaluation for Referral

Patients who are extremely hyperactive can be difficult to manage on a medical-surgical unit. Psychiatric consultation and subsequent transfer to the psychiatric unit may be necessary.

IV. POTENTIAL NURSING DIAGNOSES

1. Coping, ineffective individual, related to
   - disturbances of mood
   - hyperactivity
2. Self-care deficit, related to
   - poor personal hygiene
   - altered eating patterns
   - sleep disturbances
   - agitation, hyperactivity
3. Thought process, alteration in, related to
   - racing thoughts
   - delusions
   - hallucinations
4. Decision-making, impaired/ineffective, related to
   - disordered thoughts
   - agitation
   - impaired judgment

5. Impulsive coping mode or impulse-dominated state, related to
   - hyperactivity
   - agitation
   - hostility
6. Self-exhaustion state, related to
   - hyperactivity
   - altered eating patterns
   - sleep disturbances

V. SUMMARY

In conclusion, the hyperactive or manic patient can be cared for through a variety of interventions, including psychotropic medication, environmental restructuring, diet, and psychological/psychiatric approaches. Appropriate intervention requires recognition. Accurate recognition of the hyperactive patient is facilitated by the nursing staff's understanding of the causes of hyperactive behavior, careful observation of the patient's overt behaviors, and assessment of patient responsiveness to a series of nursing actions.

References

American Psychiatric Association (1980). *Diagnostic and statistical manual of mental disorders* (3rd ed.). Washington, DC: American Psychiatric Association.

Crawford, A. L., and Kilander, V. C. (1980). *Psychiatric nursing: A basic manual.* Philadelphia, F. A. Davis Company.

Kim, M. J., McFarland, G., and McLane, A. (Eds.) (1984). *Classification of nursing diagnoses: Proceedings of the Fifth National Conference.* St. Louis: C. V. Mosby.

Payne, D., and Clunn, A. (1977). *Nursing outline series, psychiatric-mental health nursing* (2nd ed., p. 81). Flushing, NY: Medical Examination Publication Company, Inc.

Taylor, C. M. (1986). *Mereness' essentials of psychiatric nursing* (12th ed.). St. Louis: C. V. Mosby.

Chapter 4

The Patient with Schizophrenia

Martha Josephine Snider

I. STATEMENT OF PURPOSE

There is no more puzzling phenomenon in nursing than that of schizophrenic behavior. Dealing with persons so affected is a demanding task and requires astute assessment and intervention skills.

The purpose of this chapter is:

- To increase the nurse's understanding of the broad spectrum of schizophrenic behavior.
- To enhance the nursing care of schizophrenic persons.

II. OVERVIEW OF SCHIZOPHRENIA

A. Description of the Illness

Schizophrenia is a term used to denote a group of serious, bizarre, and puzzling disorders. The general characteristics of the schizophrenic usually include gross distortion of and/or split with reality, withdrawal from interactional systems, and disorganization of perception, cognition, and affect.

Five formal subtypes of schizophrenia are generally acknowledged by the psychiatric community:

1. Catatonic type—which is typically characterized by alternating periods of stupor and excitement; mutism; odd motoric positions; world destruction and world reconstruction themes in delusions (false beliefs); and hallucinations (perceptions for which there are no outside physical stimuli).
2. Paranoid type—which is typically characterized by absurd fixed, false beliefs (delusions) that are not in concert with facts or reality. Hallucinations are common. Judgment and reality testing are consequently disturbed and behavior may be unpre-

dictable and occasionally dangerous. There may be less general personality disorganization and withdrawal than in other types. Paranoid patients are highly suspicious, distrustful, and fearful of others. Their resources for coping with anger are limited and their ability to relate to others is impaired.

3. Disorganized type—which is characterized by a more severe disintegration of the personality; flat, inappropriate, or silly affect; bizarre behavioral patterns and mannerisms; deficits in ability to respond to daily needs; and severe thought disorder.
4. Undifferentiated type—in which no one type is predominant. There may be confusion, perplexity, ideas of reference, delusions, hallucinations, highly disorganized thinking and behavior, and other manifestations usually associated with one or more types.
5. Residual type—in which mild or fairly benign indications are presented during remission of acute symptoms. During periods of exacerbation, withdrawal, eccentric behavior, irrational thinking, loose associations, and blunting of affect may be noted.

B. Incidence

The schizophrenic disorders occur in all societies. The estimated population at risk in the United States is about 1%. It has been estimated that there are approximately two million schizophrenic persons who are acutely disturbed at any given time, with about 15 times that many who are vulnerable to dysfunctional schizophrenic episodes.

The President's Commission on Mental Health (1978) reports that these persons constitute about one-half of the resident population in mental health facilities.

Men and women appear to be equally affected by these disorders. The highest incidence rate for males is between the ages 15 and 24 years and for females, between the ages 25 and 34 years.

C. Clinical Manifestations

It is important to note that not all symptoms occur in every schizophrenic individual. There is no single generally accepted "cardinal" sign or symptom, but rather a variable picture that is idiosyncratic and varies greatly over a period of time in the individual.

Deterioration from a previous level of functioning in work, relationships, and the activities of daily living is one of the commonly accepted major manifestations of the schizophrenias.

Disturbances in thought content are characterized by absurd

and illogical beliefs, or delusions. These fixed false beliefs may take the form of complaints that one's thoughts have been removed or controlled by some external force, or that thoughts are being inserted into the person's mind or broadcast to the environment like a radio transmission. Other bizarre beliefs might be that one has undergone grotesque bodily changes.

Disturbances in thought form are demonstrated by a loosening of associations in which ideas expressed are unrelated or only distantly related to one another. The patient shows no awareness that the topics are unrelated. The nurse can recognize this symptom by noting that little or no information has been communicated even though the patient may have been speaking at length.

Perceptual disorganization is characterized by a breakdown in information and sensorial processing so that the individual feels overwhelmed by stimuli. A more dramatic problem is the hallucinatory process, in which the individual's perceptions have no discernable stimuli. Any of the sensorial spheres—hearing, seeing, tasting, smelling, or touching—may be affected, though the auditory sphere is by far the most commonly reported.

Difficulties in affect may be characterized by blunting, inappropriateness, shallowness, or flatness. The emotion expressed may be clearly incongruent with the external situation or verbal message. For example, the patient may be laughing while relating a very sad event. A peculiar inability to experience pleasure or joy may be seen in individuals with long-standing problems.

Difficulties in determining the relationship of one's self to the environment, in both a physical and a psychosocial sense, can be observed, as well as disturbances in gender identity.

Ties to the external world are loosened to a greater or lesser extent. Withdrawal is enhanced by a preoccupation with fantasy and illogical thoughts. This particular feature is also related to some self-care deficits. To replace the real world, the patient creates a fantasy world for himself that is free of certain emotional stresses.

There are some disturbances in motor activity, such that there may be periods that range from hyperactivity to a marked decrease in activity. Some motor clumsiness is observed, as well as occasional posturing, grimacing, and other bizarre behaviors. These behaviors should be differentiated, however, from those that occur as side effects of antipsychotic medication.

Inability to carry out goal-directed activity may severely impair work and other role functions. This may be seen as a seeming lack of interest or inability to follow through on a course of action.

Schizophrenics characteristically have extreme difficulty establishing interpersonal relationships. Overly familiar gestures or behavior on the part of the nurse may generate anxiety or be misinterpreted by the patient.

Other symptoms seen in association with schizophrenia are depression; abnormal psychomotor activity, such as rocking or pacing; ritualistic behavior; magical thinking and ideas of reference in which the patient believes that the television or newspaper is giving special messages directly to him.

Schizophrenia generally has its onset in late adolescence or in adulthood prior to the age of 45. Before a patient can be given this diagnosis, symptoms must have persisted for a minimum of six months.

III. NURSING MANAGEMENT

A. Assessment

The assessment of schizophrenic individuals is difficult because of their propensities toward withdrawal, suspiciousness, peculiar verbal productions, and illogical thought processes.

Observation and interviewing skills, as well as a high tolerance for ambiguity and anxiety, are necessary attributes of the nurse during the assessment of these clients.

1. Assess the degree to which the person is able to act in ways commensurate with personal safety. Are judgment and reality testing disturbed?
2. Assess the ability to complete activities of daily living. Does the patient need prompting or special help in bathing, dressing, caring for teeth, hair, and beard? Does the patient have difficulty in task completion? Can the patient ask for assistance?
3. Assess the nature of thought processes as manifested through verbal communication. Does the patient have delusions? If present, what is the nature of the delusional system? Is it pervasive or circumscribed?
4. Assess for dissociative episodes. Does the patient feel as if he is standing outside himself watching himself or that he is two separate people?
5. Assess for loosening of associations and tangentiality. Does the patient associate ideas that are not normally related? Does he change topics rapidly? Is he able to sustain a train of thought?
6. Assess affect and mood for appropriateness to situation and range of affect. Is the patient able to respond emotionally to different situations or is his affect blunted or flat, with no emotion expressed?
7. Assess the presence or absence of hallucinations. Does the patient hear or see things that others do not hear or see? Are

there other sensorial experiences that cannot be validated with another person? Be particularly sensitive to the presence of command hallucinatory phenomena: Do voices command that the patient hurt himself or someone else?

8. Assess the degree of anxiety expressed by the patient regarding any experiences, fears, or fantasies.
9. Assess the presence or absence of support systems. Does the patient have friends? Does he express closeness or estrangement from family members? Does the patient have an occupation that provides a support system?
10. Assess the response of the patient to past and present pharmacological intervention for psychiatric symptoms. Be alert for complaints or behaviors that suggest the presence of side effects or toxicity. (See also Chapter 20, "Psychotropic Medications.")

B. Planning

The planning of nursing care for the schizophrenic patient is based on a continuing assessment of every facet of behavior. While there may be improvement in one or two areas of functioning, there may also be a corresponding level of dysfunction in other areas. The plan of care will, of course, be affected by the nurse's beliefs about the nature of the disorder.

C. Intervention

1. Prevention

   The status of what is known about the schizophrenias suggests that the role of genetic factors in its etiology cannot be denied. That the population at risk has been maintained at the same level for decades suggests that specific methods of prevention have yet to be identified for this group of disorders.

2. Treatment

   While acutely ill, the schizophrenic patient may well need the structure and security of a brief psychiatric hospitalization. The chronically ill and remitted schizophrenic may benefit from access to special programs such as day treatment, partial hospitalization, sheltered workshops, congregate living arrangements in the community, and the like. Certainly, a system to monitor the effects of a psychopharmacologic regimen should be available in any kind of mental health setting to which these persons come for services.

3. Medication: Antipsychotic agents

   The discovery of the neuroleptic drugs constituted a tremendous revolution in the treatment of psychotic individuals, and the use of specific medicinals with antipsychotic properties is a major form of treatment. It does fall within the purview of the nurse to assess the patient for side effects, salutary effects, and the warning signs of dangerous toxicity on a consistent basis. Moreover, it is noteworthy that other forms of treatment (individual, group, family, or social) are more effective when paired with an appropriate medication regimen.

The administration of neuroleptic drugs has been a major treatment method for schizophrenia for several years. Even without other methods of therapy, the use of drugs can decrease some of the more acute problems, such as hallucinations, delusions, agitation, and withdrawal, rather rapidly. It is believed, however, that the use of pharmacological preparations enhances the effectiveness of other forms of therapy. There is some evidence to suggest that the combination of drug therapy and psychosocial therapy is more effective than either type of therapy alone. Common drugs are Thorazine (chlorpromazine), Mellaril (thiothixene), and Haldol (haloperidol). (See also Chapter 20, "Psychotropic Medications.")

All the neuroleptic drugs have unwanted side effects, some of which are dangerous. The categories of common side effects include extrapyramidal symptoms and anticholinergic, cardiovascular, neurological, and metabolic/endocrinologic effects.

a. Extrapyramidal symptoms (EPS)

- Acute dystonic reaction

  This may occur shortly after treatment is begun and is characterized by bizarre, frightening, and often painful muscular contractions of the face, tongue, and extraocular muscles.

  Antiparkinsonian agents such as Artane (trihexyphenidyl), Akineton (biperiden), or Cogentin (benztropine) ought to be available and used quickly upon the presentation of symptoms.

- Pseudo-parkinsonian syndrome

  The person may, after a week or so of treatment, present masklike facies, rigid posture, slow movement, pill-rolling tremor of the fingers, and shuffling gait.

  Antiparkinsonian agents are usually administered to reverse these manifestations.

- Akathisia

  This side effect is characterized by restlessness, pacing, and inability to sit still, stand, or rest. Often, there are complaints of "jumpy legs" and a feeling of being "nervous inside."

  Akathisia may be confused with anxiety, and requires that the nurse differentiate between drug-related effects and anxiety so that either antiparkinsonian drugs or antianxiety measures can be taken. Continued complaints after an antiparkinsonian drug is given may suggest that the patient is experiencing anxiety or agitation rather than a side effect of the neuroleptic medication.

- Tardive dyskinesia

  Early signs of this response, which may appear after long-term drug use, involve the face, particularly the tongue. There may be bizarre grimacing and lip-smacking; "fly-catching" movements of the tongue may also be observed. Choreiform movements of the upper extremities may be present, as well as muscle contractions in the neck and back, and slow, athetoid movements of the limbs.

  Until recently, tardive dyskinesia was believed to be a permanent effect of long-term neuroleptic drug use. However, there is evidence that tardive dyskinesia can be reversed in some patients. The lowest effective dose of the antipsychotic agent should be given, and antiparkinsonian agents should be avoided when this condition is present. In addition, some evidence shows that a certain number of schizophrenic patients developed movement disorders prior to the discovery of psychotropic medications.

b. Autonomic nervous system effects: Enhanced anticholinergic effects such as dry mouth, constipation, blurred vision, sweating, and urinary retention may occur.

c. Cardiovascular effects: Orthostatic hypotension and tachycardia are common side effects.

d. Neurological effects: Lowered seizure threshold, sedation, and tremor may be noted.

e. Metabolic and endocrinologic effects: Changes in libido, disturbances in ejaculation and erection, gynecomastia, and menstrual irregularities can occur as consequences of psychoactive drugs.

4. Nursing Actions

   a. Develop consistency and regularity in a daily schedule. A structured environment can accomplish decreased levels of both anxiety and social isolation, and promote consistency in the patient's expectations of his external environment.

   b. Use regular interactional opportunities to assist the patient to test reality and validate experiences. Validate those perceptions that are rooted in reality. When perceptual distortions or hallucinations occur, the nurse should reassure the frightened patient and protect him from any external dangers or threats to safety that might arise from the patient's responses to hallucinations. This can be done in a gentle and supportive manner. The nurse must avoid validating those experiences that are a part of distortions of reality.

c. Provide and, when necessary, assist with the patient's activities of daily living (e.g., nutrition, elimination, hydration, personal grooming, exercise, and rest). People who are deeply involved in a private world of fantasy and inwardly directed mental activity may have some difficulty in expending energy on caring for themselves.

d. If the patient is known to experience delusions, redirect the patient to other interactional topics when delusional content is presented. Certainly the affect associated with fixed false beliefs should be acknowledged, though the ideational content itself should not be open to argument (e.g., "Mr. X, I have not given you a poison. I have given you your regular daily medication. I can see, though, that something has upset you."). Changing the topic with a brief explanation for doing so can be used. The attempt to use logic to defuse a delusional system is doomed to failure and may precipitate the use of more elaborate arguments by the patient.

e. Encourage the patient to participate in noncompetitive, diversionary activities with others to break patterns of social isolation. The patient may need help in learning to act in less disruptive ways around others, and this can be done through discussion and role-play if these methods can be tolerated (e.g., "Mr. X, when you take off your pajamas in the hall, it bothers people. You must not do that again. I will remind you about wearing clothes when necessary.").

f. Encourage the patient's efforts to communicate even when *what* is being communicated remains obscure. Interpretations of obvious messages are acceptable even if these are short of the mark (e.g., "I wonder if you mean that you are afraid of me.").

g. Use simple and specific language (e.g., bandage instead of dressing).

h. Focus on concrete, "down to earth" realities (e.g., "Today is Monday and you will go for the x-ray we discussed yesterday.").

i. Make decisions for the patient until he is able to do so for himself (e.g., "Wear the red pajamas now and you can choose another set this evening.").

j. Accept the patient's limitations and show approval of his capabilities (e.g., "I will help you ask the doctor questions about your operation. Let's talk about the things you'd like to know more about.").
k. Be honest. Keep any promises made.
l. Do not make demands that the patient cannot meet.
m. Attend to personal and physiological needs.
n. Protect the patient from destructiveness to self and others. Remove him temporarily from a group if his behavior becomes disruptive to others.
o. Provide the opportunity for some successful experiences when the patient is ready.
p. Suggestions for working with the suspicious or paranoid patient:
   - Give concise explanations. Use simple, matter-of-fact language.
   - Do not whisper or act in a secretive manner in the patient's presence.
   - Do not argue or disagree.
   - Limit any physical contact with the patient. The use of touch may be seen as a threat or assault or may be misinterpreted as a sexual advance.
   - Limit social interaction until the patient can tolerate the presence of others.
   - Be consistent.
   - Keep the patient informed of routines and procedures.
   - Avoid laughing or talking with others when the patient can see, but not hear, what is said.
   - Allow the patient to verbalize his feelings. Avoid defensive responses.
   - Refer to the patient as "Mr. ---." Do not use a first name or nickname.

D. Evaluation/Expected Outcomes

1. The nurse will:
   a. Provide a safe, nonthreatening, and cohesive environment for the patient.
   b. Function as a role model who demonstrates effective ways of communicating and reacting to the environment.
   c. Set limits on patient behaviors that are inappropriate or disruptive.
2. The patient will:
   a. Interact with staff and other patients.

b. Report decreased involvement in the hallucinating process. As time passes, the patient may eventually learn to ignore the "voices" when they occur.
c. Decrease the amount of verbal content devoted to a delusional system.
d. Meet his own physical needs consistently.
e. Express thoughts and feelings that relate to real events.
f. Take medications as prescribed.

E. Evaluation for Referral

1. Assess the degree to which the patient is able to attend to personal needs consistently. Should he present preoccupation or isolation behaviors that take precedence over caring for self, refer the patient for assistance from an appropriate community source (e.g., home health services, social services, visiting nurses, or community mental health services). Make sure that the community contact person is introduced to the patient prior to discharge.
2. Ascertain from the patient whom he will live with after discharge. Ensure that the medical regimen will be carried out either by the patient or by a caretaker (e.g., dressing changes, monitoring blood pressure, or special exercises).
3. If the patient has been on psychoactive drugs while in the hospital, ensure that these are prescribed by the attending physician at discharge *and* that the patient continues to have the medication regimen supported by the internist or surgeon, the psychiatrist, or the community mental health center.

IV. POTENTIAL NURSING DIAGNOSES

1. Social isolation, related to
   - hallucinations
   - delusions
   - illusions
   - dysfunctional interpersonal relationships
2. Thought process, alteration in, related to
   - impairment in reality testing and judgment
   - delusions
   - ideas of reference
   - disorganized and illogical thinking

3. Communication, impaired: verbal, related to
   - altered thought processes
   - delusions
   - hallucinations
   - inappropriate responses
   - bizarre behavior
4. Coping, ineffective individual, related to
   - disorganized thought processes
   - delusions
   - hallucinations
   - inappropriate emotional responses
5. Self-concept, disturbance in, related to
   - low self-esteem
   - difficulty differentiating self from the environment
6. Sensory-perceptual alteration, related to
   - hallucinations in any sensorial sphere
   - delusions
   - illusions
   - hypersensitivity to stimuli
   - altered thought processes

V. SUMMARY

In the past the schizophrenic has been described as the withdrawn patient because he relates poorly to reality, responds to stimuli in his own unique world, and has limited ability to form relationships. The nurse's primary tasks with the schizophrenic patient are to help him increase his contact with reality and to help him bridge the gap that exists between himself and others.

References

American Psychiatric Association (1987). *Diagnostic and statistical manual of mental disorders* (3rd ed.-rev.). Washington, DC: American Psychiatric Association.

Carpenito, L. J. (1983). *Nursing diagnosis: Application to clinical practice.* Philadelphia: J. B. Lippincott.

Carson, R. C., Butcher, J. N., and Coleman, J. C. (1988). *Abnormal psychology and everyday life* (8th ed.). Glenview, IL: Scott, Foresman and Company.

Lehmann, H. E., and Cancro, R. (1985). Schizophrenia: Clinical features. In H. I. Kaplan and B. J. Sadok (Eds.), *Comprehensive textbook of psychiatry/IV.* Baltimore: Williams & Wilkins.

Murray, R. B., and Huelskotter, M. M. W. (1987). *Psychiatric/mental health nursing: Giving emotional care* (2nd ed.). Englewood Cliffs, NJ: Prentice-Hall, Inc.

President's Commission on Mental Health (1978). *Report to the President.* Washington, DC: U.S. Government Printing Office.

Stuart, G. S., and Sundeen, S. J. (1987). *Principles and practices of psychiatric nursing.* St. Louis: C. V. Mosby Co.

Wilson, H. S., and Kneisl, C. R. (1983). *Psychiatric nursing* (2nd ed.). Menlo Park, CA: Addison-Wesley Publishing Co.

Chapter 5

The Patient with Post-Traumatic Stress Disorder

Steven L. Giles *Warren G. Clark*

I. STATEMENT OF PURPOSE

Patients requiring inpatient admissions on medical and surgical wards bring their entire history along with them when they come to the hospital. Often this history involves exposure to specific trauma such as combat, violence, or catastrophe. The traumatic event may have immediately preceded hospitalization or may have occurred much earlier in the patient's life.

The staff nurse is in a key position to observe and respond to behaviors secondary to trauma that may interface with the patient's optimal care. Hospital settings often recapitulate earlier trauma by placing the patient in a situation where he feels a loss of control and increased dependency. Perhaps the illness that caused the hospitalization (e.g., myocardial infarction) might be generating a traumatic stress reaction and early symptoms of post-traumatic stress disorder (PTSD). Other more specific physical reminders of earlier trauma—such as the hospital, other patients, or pain and suffering—may also be present. In these situations, the patient might experience increased emotional arousal and difficulty adapting to the health care environment.

It is important that the ward nurse understand the reasons for and be able to identify behaviors indicating that the patient might be experiencing symptoms of PTSD. In addition, it is important that the nursing staff be knowledgeable about appropriate intervention activities that would aid in appropriate patient care.

The following are definitions of key concepts used in this chapter (Figley 1985):

- Trauma—An emotional state of discomfort and stress

resulting from memories of an extraordinary catastrophic experience that shattered the survivor's sense of invulnerability to harm.

- Catastrophe—An extraordinary event or series of events that are sudden, overwhelming, and often dangerous either to one's self or to significant other(s).
- Traumatic stress reaction—A set of conscious and unconscious actions and emotions associated with dealing with the stressors of the catastrophe and the period immediately afterwards.

The goals of this chapter are to aid the nurse in:

- Identification of symptoms of PTSD as they are manifested in the medical and surgical patient.
- Developing practical strategies for assessment, management, and disposition of patients with this problem.

II. OVERVIEW OF POST-TRAUMATIC STRESS DISORDER

A. Description of the Illness

Following exposure to a "recognizable stressor that would evoke symptoms of distress in almost everyone" (American Psychiatric Association 1980), most people react in individual yet generally predictable ways. These behaviors can best be understood as part of the normal stress recovery process and should not be thought of as psychopathological. Stressors can include war, natural disasters, rape, violence, exposure to death and mutilation, personal injury, automobile accidents, and so on.

The recovery process follows the general overlapping course most frequently associated with reactions to death and dying. First, a person's reaction is characterized by shock and denial. This phase is usually followed by grief, anger, and, ideally, resolution. In the real world, the healing process is not always so well defined. We now know that it is quite common for survivors of tragedy to be affected for long periods of time and, at times, to have emotional experiences that can best be described as a re-experiencing of the traumatic event.

Normal stress recovery reactions appear to exist along the same continuum as PTSD symptoms. In fact, DSM-III recognizes two subtypes of PTSD. The first is referred to as acute PTSD and refers to a reaction occurring within six months of the trauma and with a duration of six months or less. The second is termed chronic or delayed PTSD and describes a reaction occurring more than six months after the trauma and/or one with a duration of symptoms of more than six months.

These differences are somewhat arbitrary. The delayed form of PTSD, with symptoms occurring suddenly following months or years without problems, is relatively rare but always dramatic. Presence of this condition is usually associated with a severe life stress or illness.

While not a critical issue in the nursing management of patients in a medical or surgical context, the issue of where normal reactions to traumatic stress end and where maladaptive or pathological reactions begin remains unanswered. It appears best to think of the entire range of reactions as evidence of ongoing stress recovery and to respond to the maladaptive and painful aspects with support and care.

Diagnosis of PTSD is made when evidence exists that the patient is re-experiencing the trauma through recurrent and intrusive recollections, including dreams of the event, or by acting or feeling like the event was happening again. Secondly, the patient must show evidence of an "emotional numbness" or diminished interest and involvement with his life and have a feeling of detachment and constricted affect. Finally, the patient must manifest at least two of the following: startle response, sleep disturbance, guilt about surviving, trouble concentrating, avoiding reminders, or increased symptoms in the presence of reminders.

B. Incidence

Information on the incidence and prevalence of post-traumatic stress disorder is generally based on either clinical estimates or general predictions based on what is known about traumatic experiences such as combat, catastrophes, and rape. It is important to note that sophisticated epidemiological investigation is only now beginning and it may be several years before accurate estimates are available.

There are settings, such as Veterans Administration hospitals, where the population is at high risk. Of the roughly 10 million veterans who served in the Armed Forces between 1964 and 1975 (the Vietnam era), it has been estimated that between 500,000 and 1.5 million have been affected by symptoms of PTSD. We are now finding that many combat veterans of earlier wars are best understood as PTSD victims, although many carry the more "traditional" psychiatric diagnoses such as schizophrenia, anxiety reaction, or personality disorder.

The frequency of exposure to catastrophe and abusive violence is not known. The literature on psychotherapy suggests that traumatic life events that are both acutely unsettling and have a lifetime legacy are, in fact, very common. Many are digested by a person's emotional resources rather efficiently, while others lie dormant or at least well contained and emerge unexpectedly to both patient and staff at times of severe stress, such as during hospitalization.

C. Clinical Manifestations

PTSD symptoms cover a broad range including behaviors related to emotional arousal, dysphoria, fear reactions, and substance abuse. As mentioned earlier, the actual stress of hospitalization may well serve to exacerbate symptoms. Other factors that might lead to symptom development during hospitalization include specific reminders such as the anniversary of the trauma, weather conditions, exposure to television or other news of a similar trauma, or even contact with patients having similar histories.

The following is a list of clinical manifestations that may be observed on a medical or surgical ward.

1. Emotional arousal

   The patient may experience a dramatic increase in generalized anxiety. This may include hyperalertness, startle response, and difficulty separating from family members. The patient may also have trouble concentrating and thus have problems adjusting to the ward environment. Anger and uncooperativeness can also be a part of the patient's presentation.

2. Dysphoria

   The patient may present as depressed and withdrawn. Crying and guilt may be manifest. Active grieving is frequently a part of the picture when the traumatic event was recent.

3. Fear reactions

   Specific fears may be noticed. The patient may refuse anesthesia or may actively fear that he is dying. The latter may appear as suspiciousness with unusual demands for explanations and education. Sleep problems are frequent; the patient may experience nightmares or exhibit a sleep phobia. A patient might have exaggerated concerns about his personal safety and security of the premises and express specific demands related to access, windows, height of the building, and so on.

4. Substance abuse

   The nurse should be particularly concerned about identifying behaviors related to substance abuse.

   An understanding of the clinical manifestations is necessary to plan appropriate nursing care for the medical or surgical patient exhibiting symptoms of PTSD.

III. NURSING MANAGEMENT

A. Assessment

DSM-III criteria appear fairly straightforward, and in many patients symptoms are quite evident. However, the assessment is complicated by the effects of certain mental mechanisms on the patient's expression of thoughts and feelings. Repression and denial help patients to manage the emotional impact of trauma, with the result of decreased overt symptoms. Guilt that results from having survived or from perceived personal responsibility may cause patients to try to hide symptoms and even to distort the existence of the traumatic event. In addition, the signs of PTSD are very often masked by other problems, particularly drug and alcohol abuse. Alcohol and other drugs often have proven helpful in masking sleep problems, flashback phenomena, and the debilitating effects of depression. Delayed PTSD is often due to prolonged self-treatment with illicit drugs.

Assessment of PTSD patients is further complicated by the fact that some patients present with "false positive" findings. PTSD can provide an excuse for inappropriate impulsive behavior on the part of the patient. Some patients choose to present themselves as victims in order to fill a desperate need for sympathy. The nurse must keep in mind the possibility of such secondary gain on the part of patients when assessing for PTSD.

The general hospital nurse assessing the patient for PTSD should be particularly alert for problems in the following areas:

1. Sleep disturbance

   The patient's sleep routine should be observed for adequate duration, restlessness, awakenings, nightmares, and so on. In addition, the sleep pattern should be observed for classic signs of anxiety or depression (onset insomnia or terminal insomnia). In the case of sleep phobia, the patient will avoid sleep at night and often look for daytime opportunities to sleep.

   When the patient experiences a nightmare, the nurse should be available to discuss the content of the dream and feelings and fears associated with it. This should be done when the patient initiates the discussion or shows a willingness to probe content. Dream material in PTSD patients is often vivid and clearly related to the precipitating traumatic event. The nurse should be cautious not to heighten the patient's anxiety by forcing a discussion or by relating dreams to trauma when the patient is denying the connection.

   Finally, the nurse should keep in mind that these patients startle easily, even while asleep. If the patient has been diagnosed as having PTSD, he should be awakened cautiously, according to his direction. This is to prevent injury related to sudden startle and to prevent undue anxiety or embarrassment for the patient.

2. Interpersonal relationships

 The PTSD patient often exhibits a severe detachment from others, even those who would be thought of as "significant others." The patient may show very little emotion toward others or conversely may show intense anger. This anger is often used as a defensive means of keeping a distance from people who might arouse memories or feelings connected with the traumatic event.

 The nurse should observe for symptoms of this detachment when families or friends visit, when the physician conducts rounds, or when the nursing staff assigned to the patient reports difficulty in establishing rapport.

 In some instances a patient may demonstrate an exaggerated fear of separation and insist on constant contact and support from family or other significant persons. Separation may act as a reminder of previous losses or may activate fears of harm to loved ones.

3. Concentration

 The PTSD patient often has difficulty in concentration. This impairment may be due to frequent thought intrusion—the unwelcome, uncontrolled recollection of the traumatic event. In such cases, the patient may appear preoccupied and disinterested or he may seem anxious or even agitated. The concentration difficulty may also be related to the patient's tendency to be hyperalert to environmental stimuli (e.g., noises, odors, touch, or the sudden appearance of a strange person).

 The nurse may note concentration deficit in several ways. She may observe the patient having difficulty in completing activities of daily living even though he is apparently physically capable of doing so. The patient may have difficulty in understanding information related to reasons for hospitalization, treatment, or outcome, despite apparently adequate intellectual functioning. The patient may be observed reading but never turning a page, or watching television but being unable to recall content. If the nurse suspects a concentration deficit, she may want to observe the patient in a structural activity, such as a patient education session, to assess the ability to concentrate and complete tasks.

4. Responsiveness to the environment

 As mentioned above, the PTSD patient may have difficulty

concentrating, resulting in misinterpretation of environmental stimuli. This concentration deficit may help set the stage for startle responses. In the PTSD patient startle responses are qualitatively different from what they would be in the general population. The PTSD patient is generally startled by a noise directly related to the traumatic event (e.g., a fire victim startled by an alarm or fire truck). In addition, the patient often feels intense anxiety following the startle, even when he realizes that there is no threat to his safety.

In its extreme form, the PTSD patient's response to the environment may take the form of flashbacks—the sudden acting or feeling as if the traumatic event were reoccurring. The nurse may note a profound change in the patient's behavior characterized in part by intense anxiety sometimes bordering on panic. In this state the patient may become disoriented and behave erratically. Flashbacks are particularly likely to occur when the patient is exposed to environmental stimuli that resemble those surrounding the initial traumatic event.

If the nurse notes problems in any of the areas noted above, she should consider that the patient may be experiencing post-traumatic stress disorder. The diagnosis can only be confirmed by a careful history taking that reveals the presence of a traumatic event and by prolonged observation for the presence of the symptoms outlined above. Diagnosis is best handled by a mental health professional. However, the observation of nursing staff can be the first indication of distress in patients reluctant to reveal the occurrence of traumatic events.

B. Planning

Planning of nursing care for the PTSD patient should be based on a comprehensive nursing assessment and subsequent nursing diagnoses, with recognition that PTSD symptoms can develop quickly. The plan should be thoroughly documented in the patient's chart and should be familiar to all nursing personnel working with the patient and family. Modification of the nursing care plan should be based on regularly scheduled reassessments of the patient's status and on evaluation of nursing care.

C. Intervention

1. Prevention

From a nursing perspective, prevention of PTSD would focus on secondary prevention or early case identification. The nurse is often the first to detect symptoms associated with both a recent traumatic stress reaction or symptoms of PTSD.

Whether a patient is involved in shock and denial of a recent stress or in re-experiencing an earlier trauma, a nurse can provide critical support that might aid in the expression of affect and assist the healing process. Grief, anger, and anxiety are exhausting for both the patient and the nurse. The nurse should be aware of her own personal resources and seek support for supervision to assist in her own affective response.

Early support and prevention can be aided by encouraging the patient to become involved in a support group or in action-oriented organizations that assist and represent survivors of specific types of trauma (e.g., veterans organizations, rape crisis centers, and victim's rights projects).

2. Treatment

   Psychotherapy is the most effective form of treatment for the patient suffering from PTSD. Through psychotherapy the survivor can begin working through and overcoming the difficult and painful emotions associated with PTSD. The successful patient often reports a sense of reintegration following therapy. In addition to specific symptom resolution, the patient will often report that his "old self" is back and his understanding of life has increased.

   "Rap groups" are a particularly effective form of therapy. These groups consist of victims of similar catastrophes and can be either self-help or professionally led.

   As mentioned earlier, victims of traumatic stress can often find solace and meaning in engaging in activities that symbolically make amends for or ensure the safety of other potential victims of trauma.

   Occasionally, inpatient psychiatric care becomes necessary when symptoms become extreme or complicated with problematic levels of substance abuse.

3. Medications

   Symptomatic treatment of depression and anxiety associated with PTSD should be short-term.

4. Nursing Actions

   As outlined above, the nurse's role in assessing the patient for problems in the areas of sleep disturbance, interpersonal relationships, concentration, and responsiveness to the environment can be critical in identifying the patient suffering from PTSD. When the diagnosis of PTSD has been established, nursing care is then based on the relevant nursing diagnosis as listed.

   a. Fear or anxiety
      - Simple reassurance and reorientation to current life circumstances can sometimes be effective. Emphasis on

safety present in the hospital setting is often a valuable patient education technique.

- Care of the anxious patient includes establishing a supportive relationship, listening, using distraction techniques, administering medications as indicated, and providing education about etiology and treatment or about controlling intrusive thoughts.

b. Ineffective coping

Nursing care depends on the specific maladaptive coping behavior being exhibited, for example:

- Flashbacks—care includes support and reorientation, avoiding confrontation, recognition of the high-anxiety state, and identifying and helping the patient avoid precipitating stimuli.
- Startle responses—care includes helping the patient identify and predict the occurrence of stimuli that elicit the startle and teaching relaxation skills to help reduce anxiety following the startle. General relaxation and stress management techniques have proved effective in reducing the intensity of the startle response.
- Referral for alcohol or drug abuse treatment as indicated.

c. Powerlessness. The nurse can help the patient gain an overall sense of confidence and self-worth that he can utilize in time of crisis by helping him identify his personal strengths, showing him respect, and allowing him to control his environment where possible. Helping him identify and either avoid or cope with situations that trigger feelings of powerlessness can also be useful.

d. Sleep pattern disturbance. Treatment of sleep pattern disturbance involves helping the patient to resolve conflicts stemming from his involvement in the traumatic event. This is usually done through psychotherapy. However, the nurse can be supportive of the patient by offering a chance to talk through his feelings while he is experiencing insomnia or following a nightmare. Other measures regarding sleep pattern disturbance were mentioned in the "Nursing Management" section.

e. Disturbance in self-concept. Again, long-range treatment of underlying guilt or inadequacy often involves psychotherapy. However, the nurse can be supportive by giving the patient honest feedback regarding his behavior, while avoiding inflating his self-esteem with false praise. Referral for psychotherapy or pastoral counseling can often be helpful in alleviating guilt. Associating with others who have been exposed to similar trauma can help the patient see that he is not alone in his suffering.

f. Potential for violence. Nursing care is essentially the same as for any violent patient and involves careful observation for behavioral cues, such as pacing, that might indicate impending violence. Violent episodes in these patients are often associated with flashbacks and are directly related to the traumatic event. The nurse must be aware that violence may occur very rapidly in these instances and that the patient may be experiencing transient gross disorientation.

   PTSD patients who demonstrate such rage reactions are generally advised to remove weapons from their homes.

D. Evaluation/Expected Outcomes

1. The measure of nursing care for the PTSD patient can be taken in two spheres:
   a. The degree to which this patient is able to complete the medical/surgical course of treatment successfully with minimal interference from PTSD symptoms.
   b. The degree to which the patient feels supported by the nurse when symptoms occur.

Measurement of each of these is highly subjective and includes data regarding sleep patterns, use of medication, methods of handling fear, anxiety and impulsivity, and the patient's self-report of well-being.

2. Expected outcomes

   In the medical and surgical nursing setting it can be expected that PTSD symptoms will diminish with resolution of the acute illness. A modification of the triggering stimuli and an opportunity for support and expression of affect should facilitate adjustment. More chronic problems, such as the nursing diagnosis of disturbance of self-concept, will not resolve in an acute treatment setting and should become part of disposition planning.

E. Evaluation for Referral

With sufficient evidence of PTSD, a treatment recommendation should always be considered following resolution of the medical illness. Patients with acute problems such as evidence of panic or potential violence should be referred for professional mental health consultation immediately. In cases where a patient is reluctant to consider referral to a mental health professional, the nurse should consider referral to an appropriate victim support group.

IV. POTENTIAL NURSING DIAGNOSES (Carpenito, 1983)

1. Fear or anxiety, related to recurrent intrusive thoughts or previous traumatic experience
2. Ineffective coping (specify flashbacks, drug use, depressions, startle responses), related to unresolved feelings (guilt, shame, anxiety) regarding traumatic event
3. Powerlessness, related to previous (sometimes prolonged) exposure to situations of helplessness
4. Self-concept, disturbance in, related to chronic feelings of guilt or inadequacy
5. Sleep pattern disturbance (nightmares), related to unresolved conflict regarding precipitating trauma or patient's exposure to trauma
6. Sleep pattern disturbance (insomnia), related to chronic depression or anxiety, drug withdrawal, fear of nightmares
7. Violence, potential for, related to impulsive expression of repressed rage associated with traumatic event

V. SUMMARY

This chapter has attempted to describe post-traumatic stress disorder as it may appear in a patient being treated for any illness. Clinical manifestations were presented and related assessment techniques were discussed. The nurse is urged to consider post-traumatic stress disorder as a possible etiology for sleep disturbances, dysphoria, disturbed interpersonal relationships, and substance abuse.

The nurse has a critical role in observing patients for these symptoms and can be a valuable resource in case finding and referral for diagnosis, psychotherapy, or support group contacts. In addition, the nurse plays an important role in supporting the patient to alleviate the effects of post-traumatic stress on the patient's concurrent health problems.

References

Adams, M. L. (1982). PTSD: An inpatient. *American Journal of Nursing, 82*(11).

American Psychiatric Association (1980). *Diagnostic and statistical manual of mental disorders* (3rd ed.). Washington, DC: American Psychiatric Association.

Berman, S., Price, S., and Gusman, F. (1982). An inpatient program for Vietnam combat veterans in a Veterans Administration Hospital. *Hospital and Community Psychiatry, 33*(11).

Carpenito, L. J. (1983). *Nursing diagnosis: Application to clinical practice.* Philadelphia: J. B. Lippincott.
Figley, C. (1985). *Trauma and its wake.* New York: Braumer/Mazel.
Furey, O. A. (1982). For some the war rages on. *American Journal of Nursing, 82*(11).
Huppenbauer, S. (1982). PTSD, A portrait of the problem. *American Journal of Nursing, 82*(11).
Keltner, N. L., Doggerr, R., and Johnson, R. (1983). For the Vietnam veteran the war goes on. *Perspectives in Psychiatric Care, 21*(3).
Mullis, M. R. (1984). Vietnam, the human fallout. *Journal of Psychosocial Nursing, 22*(2).
Norman, E. M. (1982). PTSD, the victims. *American Journal of Nursing, 82*(11).
Woods, G. C., Sherwood, T. A., and Thompson, R. M. (1985). Management and implementation of nursing care for the post traumatic stress disorder patient. In W. E. Kelly (Ed.), *Post traumatic stress disorder and the war veteran patient.* New York: Brewer Megel.

Chapter 6

The Patient with Brain Dysfunction

Jeanne DeVos

I. STATEMENT OF PURPOSE

Thinking and reasoning are so highly valued in American society that any type of brain dysfunction critically affects the quality of life. Brain dysfunction occurs more often in general hospital patients than is commonly recognized. Physical risk and psychological discomfort may occur when the significance of behaviors associated with brain dysfunction are not identified or are dismissed as "senility." Astute nursing care can decrease the threat of injury and reverse disturbing symptoms.

This chapter is designed to assist the nurse in the following ways:

- To increase understanding of the dynamics of behavior related to brain dysfunction.
- To utilize the nursing process in the management of patients experiencing brain dysfunction.

II. OVERVIEW OF BRAIN DYSFUNCTION

A. Description of the Illness

As a general term, brain dysfunction applies to a cluster of associated symptoms caused by physical or physiological impairment in functioning of the brain that results in emotional or intellectual changes in a person's mental state and behavioral patterns. Depending on the cause of the brain dysfunction, symptoms may appear episodically or continuously, and be either acute or chronic in nature.

There are numerous causes of brain dysfunction. Richard Goldberg (1980) suggests an easy-to-remember classification system for etiologies called "Mend a Mind."

M Metabolic disorder (including endocrine gland disorders and electrolyte imbalance)
E Electrical (convulsive) disorder
N Neoplastic disease
D Degenerative (chronic) brain disease (irreversible)
A Arterial (cerebrovascular) disease
M Mechanical disease (disease or injury of the actual brain structure)
I Infectious disease (e.g., AIDS)
N Nutritional disease
D Drug toxicity

It is helpful to describe the illness of the patient experiencing brain dysfunction in terms of the underlying symptom, such as confusion. Confusion may be due to systemic factors that prevent adequate cerebral support in terms of oxygen supply, nutrients, temperature regulation, control of fluid and electrolyte balance, and hydration; mechanical problems that cause obstruction to vascular flow; and untreatable irreversible dementias whose etiologies are still unclear. For the older adult in particular, consideration should be given to confusion secondary to problems of sensation and perception, social and physical environmental factors, and altered physiological states such as pain, fatigue, inactivity, and problems of elimination.

B. Incidence

Brain dysfunction can and does occur at any age and in any setting. Today the extended life span of the general population has increased the number and diversity of persons affected by brain dysfunction. Organic brain dysfunction is one of the most common reasons for disturbance in behavior. Although mental decline is often erroneously attributed to the aging process, old age is a time of increased vulnerability. Forgetfulness, altered attention, and confusion may occur more often and last longer in the older person. Often factors such as depression, social isolation, poor nutrition, and diminished hearing or vision are responsible for what appears to be intellectual decline. It is not uncommon for the older person to experience confusion secondary to chronic illness, including heart disease, cancer, stroke, and gastrointestinal disorders.

Disabling organic brain disorders increase with advancing chronological age. Alzheimer's disease, an irreversible brain disease, is the fourth leading cause of death among older Americans. About three million Americans, or about 7% of those over 65 years of age, are afflicted by this disease; it accounts for 52% of the causes of chronic brain dysfunction (Clark 1984).

C. Clinical Manifestations

Brain dysfunction may be broadly categorized into reversible and irreversible states of confusion. In *reversible brain dysfunction,* often called delirium, onset is often rapid and brief in duration. It may be associated with physical illness, trauma, or a toxic drug or substance. Reversible confusional states can also be secondary to sensory alterations and changes in the social or physical environment.

Irreversible brain dysfunction, often called dementia, is characterized by a slow, gradual onset, chronic illness, and disturbance in thinking that is severe enough to interfere with usual social and occupational activities. Both reversible and irreversible brain dysfunction produce many symptoms reflecting emotional and intellectual change. Nurses—in their strategic position of providing continuous care—are able to note the rate of change and detect variations in brain function that may make a critical difference. In the following section, clinical manifestations of both reversible and irreversible brain dysfunction are described.

Reversible brain dysfunction is manifested clinically by changes in level of consciousness that may increase or decrease wakefulness, alertness, attention, and perception of the environment. Sensory misinterpretation (illusions) or visual hallucinations may occur. Disturbed activity patterns range from agitation and restlessness to slowed movement and even stupor and coma. Often there is disorientation, first to time, then to place, and finally to person. The patient's ability to reason, make judgments, or think abstractly is markedly reduced. Frank disorder of thought, such as paranoid delusional ideation, may occur. Loss of usual social behavior may result in inappropriate undressing or impulsive acts. Although recent memory may be partially or even fully lost, remote memory of the distant past is intact. Mood is labile, with abrupt changes from laughter to tears. Anxiety is often at a severe to panic level. Speech may be incoherent. The degree of impairment related to all of the above behaviors fluctuates throughout the day, with periods of lucidity. Often the condition worsens at night, a phenomenon referred to as the "sundown syndrome."

Irreversible brain dysfunction is generally manifested by gradual changes in behavior that lead to deterioration of mental status and loss of functional capacity to meet basic needs. Early in the disease, the patient appears uncertain, indecisive, and forgetful. There may be difficulty in identifying people and hesitancy in responding to questions. Although there is a need for assistance with many activities of daily living and complaints of neglect, resentment for interference is common. Gradually the patient becomes more disoriented to time and later to place and person. Reasoning and judgment are decreased, and both recent and remote memory fail. Feelings of helplessness and of being overwhelmed often result in depression and constricted affect. As personality changes occur, periodic episodes of anxiety and fear are experienced. Later, language skills are lost, motor ability deteriorates, and the patient becomes incontinent. Death may result from infection or physiological crisis related to dehydration or malnutrition.

III. NURSING MANAGEMENT

The core of nursing management is the effective use of the nursing process, involving assessment (data collection, data analysis, and nursing diagnosis), planning, intervention, and evaluation.

A. Assessment

Data collected during the assessment process should focus on behavior interfering with the ability to function optimally and also on those strengths and resources available within the patient and the environment to promote health. Data collection in the assessment protocol suggested below is sequenced so as to provide the baseline for determining functional and dysfunctional expectations for the patient before addressing other areas such as functional status, demands for living, and resources.

1. Assess the nature and progression of the present problem.
   a. Identify the chief complaint as perceived by the patient and family.
   b. How long has the problem existed?
   c. How does it affect daily life?
   d. What coping and defense mechanisms are being used to handle the stress?
   e. What kinds of adjustments have been made from preferred or usual patterns?
2. Assess cognitive and affective function unhurriedly and after rapport has been established, realizing that the patient is often defensive and fearful. Whenever possible, ask questions conversationally so that the patient will not feel threatened. (See Appendix B for an example of a mental status exam.)

   The patient experiencing brain dysfunction may exhibit deficits in all mental status categories. The most common findings are:

a. Level of consciousness: fluctuating in reversible acute brain dysfunction, gradually deteriorating in irreversible chronic brain dysfunction
b. Mood: anxiety, fear, lability, irritability
c. Thought process: delusions, confusion, incoherence
d. Perception: illusions, visual hallucinations
e. Attention and concentration: poor
f. Reasoning: tends to be concrete
g. Judgment: poor
h. Motor coordination: poor and slow
i. Communication: brief, slow verbal responses

An organic basis for behavior must be considered whenever a patient presents with symptoms meeting one or more of the following criteria: (1) disorientation, (2) fluctuating mental status, (3) abnormal autonomic signs such as dry mouth, blurred vision, constipation, and urinary hesitance or retention, and (4) over 40 years of age with no previous history of dementia.

Although the degree of change yielded by comparison of results of tests, scales, and other assessment indicators gives significant information about patient status, it is always important to consider the patient's degree of vulnerability in terms of sensitivity to medication, sensory deprivation, or other complicating factors. Tests provide only a gross measure of change in cognitive function and should not be used alone as indicators of impairment. Of more significance to nursing is the patient's functional status and the level of support from both family and health care providers.

3. Assess physical health and health-related habits.
   a. Review the medical history and physical examination reports. Identify current medical problems. Note the type and duration of prior hospitalizations.
   b. Perform a nursing history and nursing assessment.
   c. List all medications, including name, route, frequency, and duration of all prescription and nonprescription drugs (e.g., aspirin, antacids, and laxatives).
   d. Determine use/abuse of substances such as alcohol, nicotine, caffeine, and illicit drugs.
   e. Note pain and pain relief measures.
   f. What are the usual sleeping patterns? Have there been any changes since illness?
   g. What are the nutritional patterns? What are the patient's food preferences or special diets? Is there a history of allergies, change in appetite, weight gain/loss, difficulty

chewing/swallowing, nausea/vomiting, or pain? Note the patient's fluid intake and state of hydration, ability to express thirst and to obtain fluids, and medications that affect intake and output.

h. What are the elimination patterns? Urinary: incontinence, burning/itching, frequency, hematuria, or use of a catheter. Bowel: incontinence, constipation, diarrhea, bleeding, preoccupation with excretion, or use of laxatives.
i. Have there been changes in sexual functioning (lesions, discharge, pain, menstruation, menopause, or impotence)?
j. What is the patient's energy level?
k. Determine the sensory function for vision, hearing, touch, taste, and smell. If deficits are identified, are there assisting devices (e.g., glasses, hearing aids, or dentures)?

4. Assess the level of functioning in relation to the usual and preferred activities of daily living. Focus on the patient's strengths and goals to maintain a desired lifestyle. For example, assess internal resources such as knowledge, skill, ability to communicate, values, health beliefs, and hopes. Also identify the status of external resources such as social support systems (friends, family, community, and government) and the environment (housing, transportation, shopping, and recreational facilities) (Carnevali 1984).

   At the same time that functional assessment observations are being made, the nurse may encourage, suggest, and demonstrate how the activities might be performed more effectively. The nurse should communicate to other staff and family caregivers the patient's level of independence-dependence:
   a. Independent (performs without assistance)
   b. Minimal assistance (supervision needed)
   c. Moderate assistance (aid of one required)
   d. Maximum assistance (aid of two required)
   e. Dependent (unable to help self) (Eliopoulos 1984)
5. Functional assessment factors that have the greatest potential for determining mental and emotional health include:
   a. Mobility and independence
   b. Self-care potential in performance of activities of daily living
   c. Sensory activities
   d. Ability to chew and maintain nutrition
   e. Strength to grasp hand and open bottles
6. Assess stressors and the patient's response to stress. Common stresses experienced by the patient with brain dysfunction are:
   a. Limited access to activities and health care due to disability, cost, fear, distance, transportation

b. Preoccupation with inner life as outer life decreases
c. Boredom, inactivity
d. Loss of significance, loneliness, isolation, rejection
e. Object of prejudicial treatment because of cognitive dysfunction or ageism
f. Fear of losing control, independence, concern from others, respect, dignity
g. Fear of death
h. Sense of failure, lowered self-esteem, feeling of powerlessness
i. Decrease in strength acuity
j. Diminished sensory acuity
k. Lack of closeness, intimacy, sexual satisfaction
l. Undesirable side effects of medication
m. Relocation; loss of privacy; loss of favorite belongings, food, and familiar faces
n. Limited financial resources due to inflation, cost of living, insurance, health care
o. Vulnerability to abuse from neglect or theft

Added to the above are all of the biophysiological stressors that influence thinking and psychosocial function.

7. Assess coping patterns in use at this time and those used earlier in life for dealing with stress.
8. Assess self-expectations as a demand of daily living.
9. Assess those expectations of family, friends, and health care providers that place demands upon the patient. Are expectations realistic? Is there a need for education or advocacy?
10. Assess factors in the environment or qualities of the patient's cognitive functional status that endanger the patient or present a hazard to the safety of others.
11. Assess self-concept in relation to body image, self-esteem, role performance/conflict and identity.
12. Assess resources available to the patient such as transportation community agencies.

B. Planning

Planning of nursing care is based on the identified problem and proposed etiological statement in each diagnosis. Patient-centered goals are designed to achieve measurable outcomes within a given time frame, and goal-specific nursing actions are then taken to implement the plan.

To ensure the success of planning:

1. Include the patient and family in planning by helping them determine the implications of plans and encouraging them to ask meaningful questions.

2. Make plans appropriate to both the developmental and the functional levels of the patient.
3. Formulate short-term and long-term goals that are as specific as possible and include measurable outcome criteria.
4. Identify available resources for intervention approaches to be used.

C. Intervention

1. Prevention

Prevention of organic brain dysfucntion is a multifaceted problem involving physical, psychosocial, and environmental factors. As such, it is a major personal, professional, and public concern. From a nursing perspective it is necessary to identify etiological factors clearly and to differentiate between reversible and irreversible brain dysfunction. Astute nursing observation with early detection and prompt communication of findings to other health care providers is a major means of prevention.

At present, prevention measures applicable to nursing practice include:

a. Crisis intervention
b. Suicide prevention
c. Intervention in alcohol and drug abuse
d. Public, occupational, and school health education and safety
e. Participation in immunization programs
f. Community health case finding among the lonely and isolated
g. Counseling those with a lack of understanding about medications and treatments; devising medication time tables and treatment schedules
h. Maintaining adequate nutrition; adapting special diets to accommodate cultural and ethnic health beliefs and preferences
i. Taking persistent and informed individual and group social and political action related to environmental pollution, consumer produce safety, transportation and highway safety, control of harmful substances, and occupational health and safety
j. Monitoring individuals with a history of head trauma, seizures, or cardiovascular accidents

Another area where nurses can exercise preventive action is in the anticipation and prevention of problems in people at risk:

a. Age of over 80 years
b. Sensory deprivation or overload
c. Living alone, lack of social supports
d. Confinement, especially to a horizontal position in bed
e. Relocation, especially if unplanned, sudden, and rapid
f. Unmet physical needs, especially those for ventilation, temperature control, nutrition and fluids, and freedom from pain and discomfort
g. Loss of control: sensory deficit, bowel and bladder incontinence, intubation, or restraints
h. Disruption of patterns of daily living, especially disruption in sleep cycle
i. Lack of contact with caring people
j. Loss of sense of self and the continuity of life
k. Amnesia as a result of drugs (sedatives, hypnotics, or analgesics), surgery, or trauma
l. Emotional stress

2. Treatment

The nurse plays a major role in the early detection of changes in patient status by careful and thorough assessment, accurate recording of observations, and communication of findings to other members of the health care team responsible for the prompt diagnosis and treatment of organic brain dysfunctional states. In situations involving acute, reversible brain dysfunction, the nurse supports medical treatment of the underlying pathophysiology, providing explanations and assisting the patient to adjust expectations and adapt to temporary deficits during the often uneven and slow recuperative period. Explanations to family members are also important so that it is clearly understood that the patient's disturbed behavior is temporary and that the patient is not "losing his mind" or "going crazy." If the brain dysfunction is irreversible, the nursing focus is on maintenance of biophysiological functioning, reality orientation, protection, encouragement in performing the activities of daily living, and preservation of meaningful relationships with significant others.

When brain dysfunction is acute and reversible, acute care hospitalization is generally required. If brain dysfunction is chronic and irreversible, a comfortable home environment or care by familiar, consistent staff within a long-term care facility may be more satisfactory.

3. Medications

Chemotherapy is among the most frequently used medical interventions for brain dysfunction. Drugs are etiology-specific in the treatment of acute brain disorders, for example, antibiotics for infections, hormones for endocrine dysfunction, cardiotonics and vasodilators for heart disease, and so forth, depending on the systemic disorder. Sometimes medications themselves are the cause of acute confusional states, with actions, interactions, and reactions being particularly problematic in older adults. Often, elderly patients self-medicate with over-the-counter drugs that have side effects or interact with other medications. It is crucial to identify *all* medications the patient is taking. Withdrawal of a drug or a reduction in dosage may be indicated.

Drugs used for chronic brain dysfunction basically fall into three categories:

a. Vasodilator and anticoagulants are used to increase cerebral blood flow. Because of the possibility of hemorrhage, close monitoring of blood levels and close health supervision are necessary. For homebound patients, family education and consultation with community health nurses are important.
b. Psychotropic agents are used to relieve a variety of symptoms. Antipsychotic drugs such as Haldol, Mellaril, and Thorazine may be used to lessen agitation, aggression, and thought disorder. Antianxiety drugs are used to reduce restlessness and anxiety and have even been found helpful in the relief of insomnia. For patients exhibiting apathy and lethargy, caffeine is more satisfactory than other more aggravation-producing psychostimulants. Depression, which often mimics chronic organic brain dysfunction, is significantly relieved by antidepressants. The use of all psychotropic drugs must be carefully monitored. Older adults, in particular, are at high risk for toxic side effects such as postural hypotension and tardive dyskinesia.
c. Researchers are continuously investigating new drugs. Substitute therapy, using choline and levodopa, are presently being evaluated. (*Note*: levodopa can cause side effects of paranoia or sexual acting-out in some patients.) Chelating agents are being used to bind aluminum and eliminate it from the body.

Although the success of drugs in improving behavior is variable, drugs in the last category offer new hope for the future.

4. Nursing Actions

For the patient experiencing acute brain dysfunction, reversal or partial reversal of physical symptoms can be expected to enhance the ability to cope with life and adapt to the environment. For the patient with chronic, irreversible brain dysfunction, progressive deterioration is a necessary consideration. Maintaining the patient at his most favorable level of functioning while taking into consideration his best efforts in a given situation is important.

a. Establish and maintain a high-support, low-demand therapeutic relationship.
   - Show unconditional acceptance of the patient and family members as people of human worth.
   - Build trust by being open, honest, and consistent.
   - Demonstrate empathy.
   - Confirm human dignity by showing respect.
   - Be genuinely caring.

b. Nonverbal communication is critically important; the patient may mirror the effect of those around him.
   - Offer your personal presence.
   - Sit down, be calm and relaxed (maybe quiet).
   - Have an open, friendly, warm facial expression.
   - Use direct eye contact.
   - Modulate your tone of voice to be clear, low-pitched, and steady.
   - Listen to both verbal and nonverbal communication.
   - Use a gentle, soothing, supportive touch and a firm grasp; avoid quick, startling, or hurried movements.

c. Verbal communication is a major means of interacting with the patient, his family, and others.
   - Identify yourself and call the patient by name. Ask him how he prefers to be addressed.
   - Speak to the patient, even if he appears not to be listening.
   - Talk slowly and deliberately.
   - Say one thing at a time; use short, simple sentences or a single word.
   - When repeating, repeat exactly as you first stated.
   - Avoid asking the patient too many questions; wait for a response.
   - Keep expectations and demands within the patient's capability; recognize achievements.
   - Avoid creating situations in which the patient feels he is in competition with others.
   - Avoid scolding, threatening, punishing, or rejection.
   - Remind the patient of what it is to be done.
   - Be concrete.
   - Don't refute the patient's feelings of anger, pain, or discomfort, thus minimizing them.
   - Set limits clearly and consistently.
   - Chart those phrases and techniques that work.

d. Protect the patient from injury. If there are sensory deficits, perceptual disorders, hostile/agitated behaviors, the patient is especially at risk. Safety measures include:
   - Frequent observation
   - Locked doors
   - Use of identification bracelets
   - Secure storage of medications and toxic substances; supervised administration of medication
   - Use of guard rails, side rails, and carpeting
   - Adequate lighting
   - Removal of hazards (slippery floors, obstacles, electrical equipment, and articles that could be swallowed)
   - Supervised cigarette smoking
   - Secured tubing
   - Prevention of infection
   - Prevention of hyperthermia and hypothermia
   - Help with walking and transfer
   - Assistive devices such as eyeglasses, hearing aids, and walkers, as indicated

e. Assist the patient with activities of daily living that promote health. Intellectual symptoms tend to clear slowly and unevenly. Assumption of responsibility and control should focus first upon routine activities, especially those related to personal hygiene and grooming. Patience is required by the nurse and family. Step-by-step direction about what to do and how to do it will increase the likelihood that essential tasks will be undertaken by the patient. Take the following nursing actions.
   - Ensure sufficient nutritional and fluid intake:
     - Stimulate appetite with attractive, tasty foods served in small, frequent servings. Include favorite foods and beverages. Feed the patient if necessary.
     - Offer fluids frequently.
     - Give high-calorie finger foods to hyperactive patients.
     - Prevent aspiration of foods in late stages of irreversible brain dysfunction.
     - Provide nasogastric tube feedings if necessary.
   - Maintain dentition and healthy gums through meticulous oral hygiene.
   - Assist with bathing and personal hygienic care, but encourage self-participation when the patient is able. Give special attention to appearance and grooming to facilitate social acceptance. Social acceptance will prevent social isolation, rejection, and abandonment.

- Maintain bowel and bladder elimination by consistent toileting routines; avoid invasive devices for maintaining continence (Foley catheters) if at all possible. For incontinence, if possible use external urinary devices or absorbent bed pads and change frequently; maintain cleanliness to prevent infection and skin breakdown. For regular bowel elimination, encourage a high-fiber diet, plenty of fluids, exercise, and the use of stool softeners by physician's order. Keep written records or flow sheets to determine and maintain patterns of elimination.
- Provide daily activity and exercise, keeping the patient ambulatory as long as possible (e.g., walks in the fresh air and sunshine). If the patient is bedfast, change his position frequently and perform range-of-motion exercises several times daily.
- Assist in the selection of clothing appropriate to the season or occasion, making sure that the clothing is clean.
- Capitalize on the patient's most productive periods, when his energy level is high. Help the patient conserve energy by maintaining his health status and preventing exhaustion.
- Provide adequate rest and sleep. Note disturbances, such as insomnia or wandering behaviors, requiring special attention.
- Support some withdrawal from stressful activities, particularly for the patient with irreversible brain dysfunction.

f. For the patient with altered mental status who is finding the demands of daily living overwhelming, lessen the impact of disability and facilitate adaptation to the environment. Take nursing actions to reduce anxiety and increase orientation to time, place, and person.
   - Ensure a stable, familiar, dependent environment.
   - Avoid changing routines; make changes slowly and prepare the patient for change.
   - Provide consistent care-givers and limit their numbers.
   - Provide schedules that coincide with the patient's existing habits and lifestyle patterns; simplify and structure tasks.
   - Use personal clothing and possessions.
   - Remind the patient frequently where he is and what is expected of him.
   - Provide bold-faced clocks and calendars; open the curtains during the day, turn on the lights at night.
   - Talk about what day it is and what news items are current, if appropriate.

- Use more than one sense (sensory reinforcement) to communicate a message. For example, use visual charts and color coding; reinforce verbal instructions with written instructions; utilize sound cues such as buzzers and bells; provide opportunities to taste and touch to reinforce the shape, texture, and location of objects; and accompany verbal messages with nonverbal signals or cues (e.g., asking "Do you need to use the bedpan?" and showing the pan to the patient).
- Protect the patient from confusing and threatening stimuli: bright lights, unidentifiable noises, unfamiliar faces, abstract designs on fabrics or pictures, and continuous complex communications.
- Reframe fearful situations by using new images of the problem.
- Help the patient identify precipitants to anxiety and reduce sources of anxiety.
- Provide meaningful work and physical activity to alleviate tension, boredom, and feelings of worthlessness.
- Teach relaxation techniques: slow deep breathing and progressive muscle relaxation. (For a discussion of these see Chapter 2, "The Patient with Anxiety.")

g. Assist the patient in meeting the demands of daily living by maintaining the patient's ability to live at home or in the least restrictive environment as long as possible. Family assistance and supportive community services are usually needed for activities such as paying bills, shopping, transportation, and the administration of medications. Interventions that reduce personal demands, such as housekeeping services, laundry services, beauty and barber shop services, and meals-on-wheels, are helpful. For activities that may be potentially hazardous, such as smoking or using the stove or electrical appliances, supervision should be provided.

h. One of the greatest challenges to the nurse is when the behaviors of the patient experiencing brain dysfunction seem out of control. To gain control presents a crucial challenge to daily living for the patient. Nursing actions for intervention include the following:

- Avoid confrontations with the patient who is acutely delirious and out of control as a result of disordered thought and perceptual processes. Remain nearby but do not touch the patient. Use calm, nonverbal methods such as a nod to acknowledge his statements and behavior.

The patient is usually able to remember later the events that occurred during delirium.

- Encourage the patient to recall and express feelings about disturbing episodes experienced during the time of acute illness. The release of these unpleasant emotions, accompanied by a reassurance that such reactions are common during times of illness of the type experienced, will greatly diminish frightening nightmares and persistent fears.
- Prevent agitation and screaming behavior at night by reducing fear. Help the patient gain control of the environment by providing a light in the room, an opportunity to express feelings, and the presence of a supporting person who uses a gentle, soothing touch and a calm, low-pitched voice.
- Avert evening confusion and "catastrophic" reactions in severely confused and/or cognitively impaired patients by preventing fatigue, overstimulation, and unrealistic expectations. Since the patient cannot control his behavior, there should be no penalty, expression of irritation, or withdrawal of care. Provide comfort measures, meet toileting needs, and avoid giving sedatives and hypnotics when possible.

i. Anticipate emotional reactions by noting restlessness, negativism, and a flushed face. As much as possible, avoid precipitating situations. Should the patient become agitated, hostile, and combative:

- Withdraw him to a quiet room to allow him time to calm down.
- Stay quietly with the patient. Listen.
- Use distractions such as snacks or walks.
- Avoid arguments and conflict.
- If behavior cannot be controlled with psychological measures, administer prescribed medication in low dosages. Antianxiety and antipsychotic drugs are most helpful. Avoid the use of central nervous system depressants, which often rapidly increase confusion or cause excitement.
- Avoid mechanical restraints whenever feasible. Use restraints only when necessary for safety or as a temporary measure to protect the patient until medication has brought the patient to the place where there is no longer danger to self or others. Restraints should be referred to as safety devices and applied with a careful explanation of their safety function. Privacy is important during times

of restraint. During the period of restraint there should be frequent, and periodic, scheduled monitoring of the patient, and the restrained part should be released for exercises at least every two hours. When restraints are discontinued, release should be at gradual intervals until adaptation is achieved.

j. Help the patient demonstrating frustration and anger to recognize his feelings and express them verbally in ways not destructive to himself or others. Accept the patient's use of anger as a possible effort to combat despair or make meaningful the difficulties of crisis or loss.
k. Avoid trivializing the patient's distress by insisting that he maintain a positive mood.
l. Relieve loneliness and social isolation by providing supportive interpersonal relationships, encouraging visits and letters from family and friends, and introducing diversional activities of interest. Mutual trust and compassion may be shared with a pet animal, if allowed.
m. Use the patient's own inner strengths and resources to enhance his quality of life. For example, the patient whose lifelong patterns of behavior have been optimistic, witty, and practical may respond to his illness in an easy-going manner and with a sense of humor. As a result, he may expend great efforts toward maintaining independence without being overcome by discouragement, anger, and bitterness. In contrast, if the patient is sensitive, perfectionistic, and self-sacrificing, he may tend toward withdrawal and depression. With the nurse's assistance, the patient may be helped to reach out in meaningful ways to bring pleasure to others in order to alleviate feelings of worthlessness.
n. Provide tasks or work that result in a sense of accomplishment, feelings of satisfaction, and increased self-esteem. Help the patient maintain accustomed roles, interests, and skills for as long as possible. Reinforce the patient's independence.
o. Facilitate decision making and personal control by limiting the number of choices the patient faces.
p. Avoid labeling the patient as "senile," "unreachable," or "hopeless." If the patient perceives himself as a passive victim or the recipient "object" of service, the loss of a sense of identity and meaning to life results in a spiraling process that leads to vegetation and death (Ebersole and Hess 1985).

q. Inspire hope by helping the patient draw upon personal resources and sustaining relationships with loved ones. The nurse may say, "Tell me about your wife and some joyous experiences you've shared." If the patient is unresponsive, repeating the loved one's name, playing familiar favorite music, or demonstrating the use of touch and closeness will foster meaningful, life-promoting bonds. When loved ones are present, the nurse should ensure that privacy is provided for precious times of closeness (Miller 1985).
r. Be open to expressions of spiritual need or belief. Often the strongest sources of hope and comfort are the patient's faith and hope in God.
s. Make real the qualities the patient needs when facilitating his efforts to realize spiritual health.
t. Refer the patient to a member of the clergy as needed or upon request.
u. Make sure that social stimulation is meaningful to the patient. Prevent overload and complex activities; mildly stimulating activities or experiences are best. For example, aesthetic senses may be enhanced with pleasant aromas, colors, pictures, plants, or textured surfaces. Both life satisfaction and social interaction may be increased through a broad range of creative artistic programs utilizing techniques of art, music, dance, and poetry or prose.
v. Work with the family and significant others as an external resource whose influence and decision making will be a major determinant in the long-term outcomes for the patient.
   - Assist in the development of realistic expectations by keeping family members well informed concerning the patient's mental and physical status, the meaning of behavior, and anticipated changes in behavior.
   - Promote a relationship with health care providers that is open, honest, and hopeful.
   - Encourage collaborative participation by the family in the nursing care planning process.
   - Teach supportive care measures to family members:
     - Basic interventions for dealing with activities and demands of daily living
     - Special procedures that the family can perform
     - Ways to prevent problems
     - How to respond to problematic behaviors
     - Supervision of safety
     - Ways of maintaining the patient's interests and skills

- Support the delivery of care by being a resource person to answer questions and provide information.
- Explain the patient's need for independence to enhance self-esteem.
- Prepare the family as well as the patient for diagnostic tests:
    - Explain the test and behavior expected from the patient in simple terms.
    - Answer questions and repeat explanations just before the test.
    - Help the family obtain correct and timely written information.
    - Provide emotional support and personal presence at the time.
- Support the family through reinforcement, recognition, and counseling:
    - Help the family not to personalize what the patient says or does.
    - Encourage expression of concerns, needs, and feelings. Listen.
    - Urge family members to take care of their own nutritional, leisure, and rest needs.
    - Discuss strategies for adjustment of family roles.
    - Explain the process of grieving as a normal response to loss. Assist the family through the grieving process.
    - Allow family members to express anger about the difficulties of care giving and demands placed on them.
    - Identify coping strategies for dealing with frustration and anxiety.
    - Teach problem-solving skills; help the family to focus on one problem at a time.
    - Teach assertiveness skills for dealing with service agencies and the health care system.
- Utilize community support services:
    - Provide information and referral for adult day care and other respite care services.
    - Enlarge the social support network (e.g., home health agencies, equipment supply houses, church groups, and support groups with other families in similar circumstances).
    - Set up a file of personal papers.
    - Assist in obtaining legal aid.
- Express appreciation for input, care efforts, and loyalty.
- Reduce feelings of embarrassment, shame, and regret by focusing on the present instead of the past and by

encouraging active participation in adding to the patient's quality of life each day.

D. Evaluation/Expected Outcomes

Evaluation is an ongoing process to determine the effectiveness of nursing actions in helping the patient achieve health-related goals. Measurement of goal achievement is based upon outcome criteria and time frames established during the planning phase of the nursing process. As a result of evaluation, new data is generated for modification of the nursing care plan.

1. The nurse will:
   a. Provide a safe environment and protect the patient while he is disoriented (close observation, proper use of mechanical restraints when necessary, sedation as needed, bed in low position).
   b. Observe the patient closely for changes in mental status and document any changes.
   c. Support the patient with nursing interventions throughout the diagnostic process and treatment to correct any medical problems.
2. The patient will:
   a. Remain injury free during hospitalization.
   b. Maintain anxiety at a mild-to-moderate level in interactions with the care-givers by discharge.
   c. Perform activities of daily living with the assistance of the care-giver by discharge.
   d. Achieve his maximum capability of contact and interpretation of reality by discharge.
   e. Decrease memory deficit to maximum potential (recent and remote).
   f. Maintain or achieve the maxmium possible health status (weight, skin integrity, nutrition, elimination, and so on).
   g. Be free of delusions, hallucinations, and illusions by discharge.

IV. POTENTIAL NURSING DIAGNOSES

This list of possible nursing diagnoses relates to the emotional needs of patients with brain dysfunction. Nursing diagnoses related to physiological problems would also apply.

1. Anxiety (moderate), related to
   - unfamiliar environment
   - loss of control over life
   - impaired cognitive function
2. Communication, impaired verbal, related to loss of memory of language use
3. Coping, ineffective individual: depressed mood and continuous crying, related to
   - uncertainty about future
   - insecurity about economic status
4. Embarrassment related to memory loss
5. Fear, related to
   - loss of control
   - unfamiliar care-givers
   - unpredictable environment
6. Frustration, related to impaired short-term memory
7. Grieving, related to
   - loss of functional capacity in activities of daily living
   - changes in self-image
   - loss of loving relationships
8. Home maintenance management, impaired, related to
   - forgetfulness
   - loss of skill to perform tasks
9. Injury, potential for: falls, related to
   - disorientation
   - muscle weakness
   - wandering behavior
10. Powerlessness, related to unfamiliar environment
11. Self-concept, disturbance in: low self-esteem, related to increased dependence on others to perform self-care
12. Socially inappropriate aggressive behavior, related to lack of impulse control
13. Socially inappropriate behavior: undressing in public, related to misinterpretation of reality
14. Social isolation, related to
    - feelings of rejection by significant others
    - sense of abandonment
    - sense of meaninglessness to life
    - sensory deficit: hearing
    - decreased level of consciousness
    - withdrawal pattern of behavior
    - agitation

15. Spiritual distress, related to
    - unresolved guilt
    - sense of hopelessness
    - inability to forgive oneself or others

E. Evaluation for Referral

The nature of care with the patient experiencing brain dysfunction involves both acute and long-term care. Although one of the critical variables in long-term care is the family, there needs to be a balance between family responsibility and support from the formal health and community care systems (Hays 1988). To provide this support requires that nurses act not only as social welfare advocates and educators of health policy makers, but also as major referral agents. Particular services helpful to the patient and family dealing with brain dysfunction include:

1. Medical diagnostic and research centers
2. Rehabilitation centers and services
3. Day care and respite services
4. Home health agencies
5. Nursing homes
6. Community mental health centers
7. Family support groups
8. Hospices
9. Centers for independent living
10. Immunization clinics in health departments
11. Medical equipment and supply houses
12. Churches and synagogues
13. Therapeutic dietetic services
14. Physical therapy
15. Welfare and social security administration services
16. Homemaker services
17. Meals-on-wheels

V. SUMMARY

Reversible and irreversible brain dysfunction are manifested by a broad spectrum of conditions, symptoms, and behaviors. The threat and disorganization that results in the lives of patients and families calls for immediate support as well as sustained long-term relationships with health care providers. Relating to the patient and family requires patience and determination. Empathy and hope are needed to move the patient and family toward healthy coping.

Quality of life and adequate care for persons experiencing brain dysfunction are among the greatest challenges facing health care delivery systems today. Nursing is uniquely prepared to meet these challenges as it moves to the forefront among health care professionals. Trends are from high tech to high touch, from hierarchies to networking, from institutional to self-help, and from either/or to multiple options (Naisbitt 1982). Nurses work toward patient and family participation in controlling their own lives.

Nursing management for the patient with brain dysfunction is focused on a balance between activities and demands of daily living and internal and external resources. The nurse must share knowledge and skill in the systematic use of the nursing process to generate approaches that result in increased functional behaviors for the patient and family.

References

American Psychiatric Association (1987). *American Psychiatric Association: Diagnostic and statistical manual of mental disorders* (3rd ed.-rev). Washington, DC: American Psychiatric Association.

Carnevali, D. L. (1984). *Diagnostic reasoning in nursing.* Philadelphia: J. B. Lippincott.

Clark, M., et al. (1984). A slow death of the mind. *Newsweek* (December), 56–62.

Doyle, G. E., et al. (1986). Investigating tools to aid in restorative care for Alzheimers patients. *Journal of Gerontological Nursing, 12*(9), 19–24.

Ebersole, P., and Hess, P. (1985). *Toward healthy aging: Human needs and nursing response.* St. Louis: C. V. Mosby Company.

Eliopoulos, C. (1987). *Gerontological nursing.* Philadelphia: J. B. Lippincott Co.

Gillis, D. A. (1986). Patients suffering from memory loss can be taught self-care. *Geriatric Nursing, 5,* 257–261.

Goldberg, R. (1980). *Psychiatry for the primary physician.* Darien, CT, Patient Care Publications.

Hays, A. (1988). Family care: The critical cariable in community-based long-term care. *Home Healthcare Nurse, 6*(1), 8–9.

Lipowski, Z. (1980). A new look at organic brain syndrome. *American Journal of Psychiatry, 137*(6), 674–678.

Martens, K. (1986). Let's diagnose strengths, not just problems. *American Journal of Nursing, 86*(2), 192–193.

Matherson, M. A., and McConnell, E. S. (1988). *Gerontological nursing: Concepts and practice.* Philadelphia, W. B. Saunders Co.

Miller, J. F. (1985). Inspiring hope. *American Journal of Nursing, 85*(1), 22–25.

Naisbitt, J. (1982). *Megatrends: Ten new directions transforming our lives.* New York: Warner Books.

Shelly, J. A., and John, S. (1983). *Spiritual dimensions of mental health.* Downers Grove, IL: Inter Varsity Press.

Wilson, H. S., and Kneisl, C. R. (1988). *Psychiatric nursing* (3rd ed.). Menlo Park, CA: Addison-Wesley Publishing Company.

Wolanin, M. O., and Phillips, L. R. F. (1981). *Confusion: Prevention and care.* St. Louis: C. V. Mosby Company.

SECTION TWO
PERSONALITY DISORDERS

Chapter 7

The Patient with an Antisocial Personality Disorder

Giovanna B. Morton

I. STATEMENT OF PURPOSE

The nurse will frequently encounter patients who have characteristics associated with antisocial personality disorder. This chapter is designed to assist the nurse to:

- Identify common behavioral characteristics exhibited by patients with antisocial personality disorder.
- Apply the nursing process in providing care for patients with antisocial behavior characteristics.

II. OVERVIEW OF ANTISOCIAL PERSONALITY DISORDER

A. Description of the Illness

The antisocial personality disorder is one of the most fascinating and, at the same time, one of the most exasperating of all the personality disorders. The behavior of these patients has been labeled in many ways over the years from "constitutional psychopathic inferiors" to "psychopaths" to "sociopaths," indicating both the origin and the nature of the illness. Today, the Diagnostic and Statistical Manual of the American Psychiatric Association (DSM III-R) classifies this illness under "Personality Disorders," where it is called "Antisocial Personality Disorder" (APA 1987). The disorder is called "antisocial" because the behavior shown by these patients is typically in violation of laws, mores, and customs

(Janosik and Davies 1986). "Antisocial personality also refers to an aggressive behavioral pattern such as is seen in the person who "acts out" like the explorer, the soldier, the pioneer, or even the delinquent and the criminal (Johnson 1986).

In health care settings, the nurse often sees this disorder in the form of manipulative behavior and therefore these patients are referred to as "manipulative patients." No matter what label is attached to these patients, the behavior that is often seen is one that shows a lack of conscience. These patients seek immediate gratification of their needs, are unable to postpone pleasure, and are unable to tolerate delays or frustrations. Most of these patients will appear to be very charming and intelligent in order to manipulate others to help satisfy their own needs. These people usually lack concern for others and have little or no loyalty. As a consequence, they are usually unable to maintain close and lasting relationships with either persons or groups. They do not learn from experience. Punishment is rarely effective because these patients have little anxiety or guilt feelings. A common tactic used by these patients is to induce sympathy or guilt in another person to make it impossible to refuse a request. Not trusting others to meet their needs, antisocial patients manipulate rather than approach others directly. These patients frequently play one person against another and then sit back and enjoy the turmoil that they have created.

B. Incidence

How this disorder develops still remains unknown; however, it is commonly believed that genetic, constitutional, maturational, and environmental factors may play a role in the development of the antisocial personality disorder (Freedman et al. 1977).

Often there is a history of chaotic home environment, maternal deprivation in early life, and a history of little affection being shown to the child. Evidence also indicates that separation of parents and divorce, along with absence of discipline from parents, seem to foster this behavioral pattern. The fathers of those affected frequently have the same disorder. Electroencephalogram (EEG) findings in some patients show an excess of bilateral rhythmical slow-wave activity (Wilson and Kneisl 1988; Adams 1981). This seems to indicate a physiological base for this disorder in some cases.

All authorities seem to agree on the fact that the manipulative type behavior exhibited by these patients appears to be learned in childhood or adolescence from parents or significant others.

People with these behavior patterns were thought to be found primarily in delinquent and criminal circles and, therefore, this behavior problem was believed to be confined to penal institutions. In actuality, this type of personality disorder permeates all levels of business, medicine, religion, law, and government.

The worldwide incidence of this disorder is not known, but in the United States it is estimated that about 3 percent of American males and 1 percent of American females have this type of personality disorder. The onset is said to be in early childhood for males and in puberty for females (Coleman et al. 1984). This disorder is on the rise in the United States. It has been suggested that the nation has passed from an "age of anxiety" and developing "neuroses" to an "age of narcissism" and developing problems having to do with love for the "self." This is reflected in the current emphasis placed on self-gratification, self-indulgence, and self-development to the exclusion of the needs of others (Johnson 1986).

C. Clinical Manifestations

Since this disorder begins in childhood or early adolescence and affects the person in multiple life areas of social functioning, the clinical picture will vary considerably.

The typical adult characteristic symptom pattern associated with antisocial personality disorder will include five major areas, according to Coleman and colleagues (1984):

1. Inadequate conscience development and lack of anxiety and guilt. These patients accept ethical values on a verbal level but are unable to internalize this meaning. Intellectually they are normal or above normal but their conscience development is severely retarded or nonexistent. Their appearance of sincerity, combined with their lack of anxiety and guilt, many times enables them to avoid suspicion and detection for stealing and other illegal activities.
2. Irresponsible and impulsive behavior; low frustration tolerance. Antisocial patients generally have a callous disregard for the rights, needs, and well-being of others. They usually take from others rather than earn what they want. They seek adventure without regard for consequences. They live in and for the present moment, so that long-term goals are out of the question. External reality is used for immediate personal gratification. They are unable to endure routines or shoulder responsibility, so they either manipulate others to do their job or they change jobs.
3. Ability to put up "a good front" to impress and exploit others, projecting blame onto others for their own socially disap-

proved behaviors. Antisocial patients are often charming and likeable, and consequently they win friends easily. They usually have a good sense of humor and an optimistic outlook. They frequently lie and when caught express sorrow and vow to make amends but never do so. They have excellent insight into other persons' weaknesses and needs and are very skillful at exploiting them. They easily find excuses for their antisocial conduct and project the blame onto someone else. Thus, they are capable of convincing others and themselves that they are free of fault.

4. Rejection of authority and inability to profit from experience. Antisocial patients behave as if social regulations do not apply to them. No matter what difficulties their behavior may cause, they seem incapable of learning from the experience.
5. Inability to maintain good interpersonal relationships. In spite of the many friends they make, they are unable to keep them. They are irresponsible and egocentric, and ungrateful, unsympathetic, and remorseless in their dealings. They cannot understand love in others or give it in return.

III. NURSING MANAGEMENT

Effective nursing management utilizes the nursing process in the accomplishments of its goals, that is, assessment, planning, intervention, and evaluation.

A. Assessment

1. Patients with antisocial personalities use action as a primary form of expression. They also possess characteristic ways of perceiving, thinking, and feeling (Johnson 1986). The nurse needs to assess:
   a. Perception

      Antisocial personalities perceive other people and the world as harmful, hostile, and out to undermine their independence. They thus view others as a source of threat to their independence because they perceive themselves as "super independent." They see themselves as assertive, self-sufficient, competitive, powerful, and superior. Because they value these characteristics, they reject attributes associated with warmth, caring, or compassion in both themselves and others.

   b. Thinking

      Antisocial patients believe that human beings are

basically evil; therefore, they have the right to take an antagonistic stance towards others and society. This gives them the power to develop schemes and tactics to outwit and punish others.

c. Feeling

Antisocial patients are basically hostile, punitive, and vengeful people who project their weaknesses to others and therefore mistrust others. They are particularly suspicious of people who are warm and compassionate and believe that these people are out to undermine their independence.

2. The antisocial patient will express these characteristics in the following specific nonverbal and verbal behavioral patterns of which the nurse should be aware:
   a. They become easily bored, restless, and frustrated when faced with monotonous routines and responsibilities. To counteract this, they impulsively seek thrills and dangers to buffer these feelings. For example, they will become involved with fighting, aggressive sexual behavior, vandalism, outbursts of explosive anger, chemical abuse, violence, and abuse and exploitation of others.
   b. Verbal behaviors exemplified by the antisocial patients are derogatory, humiliating, and "belligerent verbalizations directed to or about persons perceived as threatening, vicious argumentation and insults, and other forms of violent, verbal abuse" (Johnson 1986). Not all behavior will be manifested in a crude, callous manner, however. Some patients will be able to be keenly aware of the moods, feelings, and weaknesses of other persons and use these to manipulate, exploit, and control others in order to acquire power and maintain their independence.

B. Planning

Planning is based on a thorough assessment of the behavior of the patient as well as on the history of the patient. According to Janosik and Davies some of the goals that should be included in the nursing care plan are to assist the patient to:

1. Become aware of his behavior in relation to others and find more appropriate ways to obtain what he needs.
2. Foster the ability to trust others to meet his needs without having to resort to manipulation and exploitation of others.
3. Live with consistent limits and expectations.
4. See the advantages of cooperation, compromise, and collaboration over antisocial or manipulative behavior.

C. Intervention

1. Prevention

The best measure to prevent antisocial personalities from developing would be to provide stable, secure, loving, mature parents who are themselves emotionally and mentally healthy. If this is not possible, it would be advantageous to provide corrective experiences for the children and adolescents who are at risk. These experiences could be provided through the school system or community mental health centers. It is imperative that the children have the opportunity to identify with adults who are warm, trusting, loving, and secure adults who can reciprocate these feelings and behaviors with the child. It is likewise important that children witness parental behavior that demonstrates respect for others as human beings and not that which "uses" or "abuses" others for personal gain.

2. Treatment

Most people with an antisocial personality disorder neither seek nor believe that they need psychiatric help; therefore, few people with this disorder will be found in mental health treatment settings. If they are hospitalized, it is usually because of some other reason.

The treatment of the antisocial patient is aimed at assisting the patient to establish controls over his behavior. This is accomplished by maintaining a firm but accepting attitude toward the patient and at the same time imposing external limitations on the behaviors of the patient. An inpatient setting may be needed to provide the necessary external controls.

The most beneficial form of treatment to date is psychotherapy. The goal of this therapy is to assist the person to gain insight into his behavior and eventually learn how to use this new insight to change his behavior.

As they age, some patients show a decrease in the range and severity of antisocial behavior. Improvement most often occurs between the ages of 30 and 40. Relationships with people seem to improve and they seem to experience less difficulty with the police (Adams 1981).

Milieu therapy has been tried and found to be fairly successful. These patients respond best to structured, controlled settings rather than loose, permissive settings (Adams 1981).

3. Medications

There are no medications to assist in the recovery of a

patient with an antisocial personality disorder. However, this disorder may occur in combination with other problems such as chemical abuse. In this case, certain medications may be indicated to assist the patient with the chemical abuse problem.

4. Nursing Actions

Should the antisocial patient be hospitalized, intervention will be more effective if the nurse takes the following actions (Johnson 1986):

a. Develops self-awareness

These patients have a cunning way of provoking other people. It is not unusual for the nurse to feel anger towards the patient, to become defensive, to desire to control the patient, and to become flustered and unable to function adequately while working with the patient. The nurse needs to accept these feelings and not act upon them. It would be wise for the nurse to talk with a trusted nurse colleague in order to increase the nurse's self-awareness and maintain emotional control.

b. Develops trust

Since antisocial patients do not trust, special care should be taken to establish trust. It is essential to maintain a matter-of-fact approach rather than a warm, friendly approach with these patients. Trust can be fostered if the nurse is punctual, honest, respectful, and genuine.

The nurse should use caution in interpreting the behavior of these patients to them, since they may view this as an act of intrusion and control. Communication should be kept open and focused on the behavior of the patient. This can best be accomplished through the use of open-ended questions, for example, "Tell me about your argument with Mr. X."

Verbal and nonverbal behavior on the part of the nurse should remain congruent, otherwise the patient will misinterpret this behavior and become suspicious of the nurse.

c. Uses confrontation

Confrontation is especially useful in working with antisocial patients who use manipulation. The purpose of confrontation (pointing out a patient's problematic behavior to him) is to assist the patient to become more self-aware of his behavior. To use confrontation effectively, the nurse should:

- Point out the behavior as soon as possible.
- Be specific in describing the behavior.

- Use a matter-of-fact, nonjudgmental manner.
- Focus on the actual behavior.

  Confrontation needs to take place in a safe and secure environment for the patient, otherwise the patient will become defensive. Before confrontation can take place, trust must exist between the patient and the nurse.

d. Sets limits

The nurse must set limits for patients who display manipulative, dependent, and acting-out behaviors. Setting limits lends security to a situation and helps to curb the behavior displayed by antisocial patients. For setting limits to be effective, the nurse must:

- Identify behavior that needs to be changed or controlled.
- Ask the patient in a matter-of-fact manner to control the behavior.
- Offer an appropriate, alternate behavior for the patient to pursue.
- Expect the patient to test the nurse to determine if the nurse will break down.
- Remain steadfast and consistent in the use of setting limits.

  When the antisocial patient is on a medical-surgical unit it may be helpful for staff to seek consultation with the psychiatric nurse clinical specialist in order to establish a plan of care that includes reasonable, but firm, limits.

D. Evaluation/Expected Outcomes

Positive evaluation is reflected in the successful fulfillment of expected outcomes or goals. If any goals have not been met, the nurse should seek to find out why. Failure to resolve a problem may rest with the patient, the nurse, or the nature of the goal.

1. The nurse will:
   a. Be constantly aware of the possibility of manipulative behavior.
   b. Establish firm but fair limits on the patient's behavior.
   c. Explain the limits (rules) clearly and early in treatment.
   d. Work with the treatment team so that all team members use a consistent approach with the patient.
   e. Help the patient learn to accept and utilize more socially acceptable attitudes and behavior in relating to others.
2. The patient will:

a. Demonstrate increased impulse control.
b. Function within the rules and limits of the treatment setting.
c. Avoid harm to self or others.
d. Identify the behavior that precipitated hospitalization.
e. Demonstrate more positive ways of coping with frustration.
f. In time, accept that it is the poor choices *he,* not others, makes, that create difficulties for him.

E. Evaluation for Referral

Success in making behavior changes in the antisocial patient is difficult and often temporary. The patient may repeatedly return to the hospital or to jail. Long-term changes in behavior can take years of therapy, and the patient must see a need for change. The patient's state of mind is a critical factor. The best time to reach the antisocial patient and refer him for treatment is when he is vulnerable. The patient may have periods when he becomes fed up with himself and has doubts about his way of life. He may be especially vulnerable to considering change when faced with a crisis such as a serious illness or incarceration, or when facing unknown consequences. The antisocial patient is rarely reached by traditional methods of therapy, but rather by long-term treatment designed to alter and restructure his patterns of thinking.

IV. POTENTIAL NURSING DIAGNOSES

1. Violent/acting out behavior (verbal/nonverbal) to release tension and/or to gain control, related to
   - disregard for feelings and rights of others
   - inability to delay gratification
   - impulsivity
   - impaired judgment
   - impaired coping ability
   - disregard for rules and regulations
2. Manipulations to gain control or for personal gain, related to
   - inability to delay gratification
   - disregard for the needs of others
   - dishonesty
   - feelings of entitlement

3. Poor impulse control, related to
   - weak ego boundaries
   - low frustration tolerance
   - poor judgment
   - inability to delay gratification
4. Ineffective social and interpersonal relationships, related to
   - excessive need for control or independence
   - excessive dependency needs
   - poor social skills
   - fear of intimacy
   - hostile or angry abusive behavior
   - inability to feel remorse
   - failure to learn from past experiences
   - disregard for rules and regulations
   - suspiciousness
   - clinging "demandingness"

V. SUMMARY

Antisocial patients have many problems even though on the surface they appear normal. The manipulative and irresponsible behavior these patients often display indicates perceived needs that they have. Their needs and behavior must be balanced with the principles of good nursing care. They constitute some of the most difficult and frustrating patients to care for, but the nurse must avoid the attitude and actions that give the impression that "This patient won't change, anyway, so why bother?" For if the nurse gives up, who will care?

References

Adams, H. E. (1981). *Abnormal psychology.* Dubuque, IA: Wm. C. Brown Company Publishers.

American Psychiatric Association (1987). *Diagnostic and statistical manual of mental disorders* (3rd ed.-rev.). Washington, DC: American Psychiatric Association.

Beck, C. M., et al. (1988). *Mental health—Psychiatric nursing.* St. Louis: C. V. Mosby Company.

Burgess, A. W. (1985). *Psychiatric nursing in the hospital and the community* (4th ed.). New Jersey: Prentice-Hall, Inc.

Coleman, J. C., Butcher, J. N., and Carson, R. C. (1984). *Abnormal psychology and modern life* (7th ed.). Glenview, IL: Scott, Foresman and Company.

Freedman, A. M., Kaplan, H. I., and Sadock, B. J. (1976). *Modern synopsis of comprehensive textbook of psychiatry II.* Baltimore: Williams & Wilkins Co.

Frosch, J. P. (1983). The treatment of antisocial and borderline personality disorders. *Hospital and Community Psychiatry, 24*(3), 243–248.

Janosik, E. H., and Davies, J. L. (1986). *Psychiatric mental health nursing.* Boston: Jones and Bartlett Publishers, Inc.

Johnson, B. S. (1986). *Psychiatric-mental health nursing: Adaptation and growth.* New York: J.B. Lippincott Company.

McMorrow, M. E. (1981). The manipulative patient. *American Journal of Nursing, 81*(6), 1189–1190.

Murray, R. B., and Huelskoetter, M. M. W. (1983). Giving emotional care. In *Psychiatric mental health nursing.* Englewood Cliffs, NJ: Prentice-Hall, Inc.

Platt-Koch, L. M. (1983). Borderline personality disorder. *American Journal of Nursing, 83*(12), 1666–1671.

Rowe, C. (1984). *An outline of psychiatry* (8th ed.). Dubuque, IA: Wm. C. Brown Company Publishers.

Wilson, H. S., and Kneisl, C. R. (1988). *Psychiatric nursing* (3rd ed.). Menlo Park, CA: Addison-Wesley Publishing Company.

Chapter 8

Patients with Other Personality Disorders

Theodore B. Feldmann

I. STATEMENT OF PURPOSE

Personality is the sum total of a person's internal and external patterns of adjustment to life. It is the repertoire of problem-solving techniques that an individual acquires during growth and development. Personality is relatively stable over time and reflects the coping mechanisms and ego defenses that an individual uses to maintain emotional equilibrium. Personality may thus be thought of as an individual's characteristic way of dealing with the world.

With the above definition of personality in mind, it becomes relatively easy to define a personality disorder. When the personality traits exhibited by an individual are inflexible or maladaptive and cause significant impairment in social or occupational functioning, a personality disorder is said to exist. These disorders are usually apparent by adolescence and remain prominent throughout adult life. We all exhibit traits of different personality disorders at different times, especially during times of extreme stress. It is important to remember that a personality disorder exists when maladaptive traits become the primary way of dealing with the world.

This chapter is designed to provide a basic introduction to personality disorders. Emphasis will be placed on the current classification system as well as the diagnostic criteria for each personality disorder. The antisocial personality disorder presents special challenges and problems, and was dealt with in Chapter 7 of this text.

II. OVERVIEW OF PERSONALITY DISORDERS

A. Description of the Problem

In recent years psychiatrists, and in particular psychoanalysts, have become increasingly interested in the personality disorders.

This results, in part, from the introduction in DSM-III, the standard for psychiatric nomenclature in the United States, of specific diagnostic criteria for the personality disorders. Previously these disorders consisted of vaguely and subjectively defined traits. As the personality disorders have become more well-defined and as theories have been developed to explain their occurrence, a greater appreciation of their frequency has emerged. In clinical practice the personality disorders are quite common. It is also recognized that many people with personality disorders never seek treatment. This is because the spectrum of symptoms displayed by these patients ranges from only mildly distressing to totally incapacitating. Generally it is only the more severe cases that come to psychiatric attention.

In general, the personality disorders may be thought of as occupying a spectrum of psychopathology lying between the neuroses and the psychoses. As would be expected, those disorders situated at the more neurotic end of the spectrum would be more adaptive and generally healthier. Those closer to the psychotic end of the spectrum show more serious signs of psychopathology, with a lower level of functioning. By viewing the personality disorders in this manner, it can be understood that the disorders closer to the neuroses would be characterized by a higher degree of ego- or self-integrity and those disorders closer to the psychotic end of the spectrum would be characterized by a tendency for ego- or self-fragmentation. Figure 8–1 illustrates this concept.

The personality disorders, as classified in DSM III-R, can be grouped into three clusters, each characterized by a typical pattern of behavior. The first cluster is characterized by odd or eccentric behavior, and includes the paranoid, schizoid, and schizotypal personalities. The next cluster is marked by dramatic, emotional, and often unpredictable behavior, and includes the histrionic, narcissistic, borderline, and antisocial personality disorders. The third cluster contains those disorders that present with prominent anxiety and fearful behavior, and consists of the avoidant, dependent, compulsive, and passive-aggressive personalities.

B. Incidence

The incidence of serious personality disorder reported in the adult population ranges from 5%–15% (Frosch 1983). Manifestations of personality disorders can often be recognized in childhood or adolescence and continue throughout most of adulthood. These traits may become less obvious by middle age or old age (American Psychiatric Association 1980).

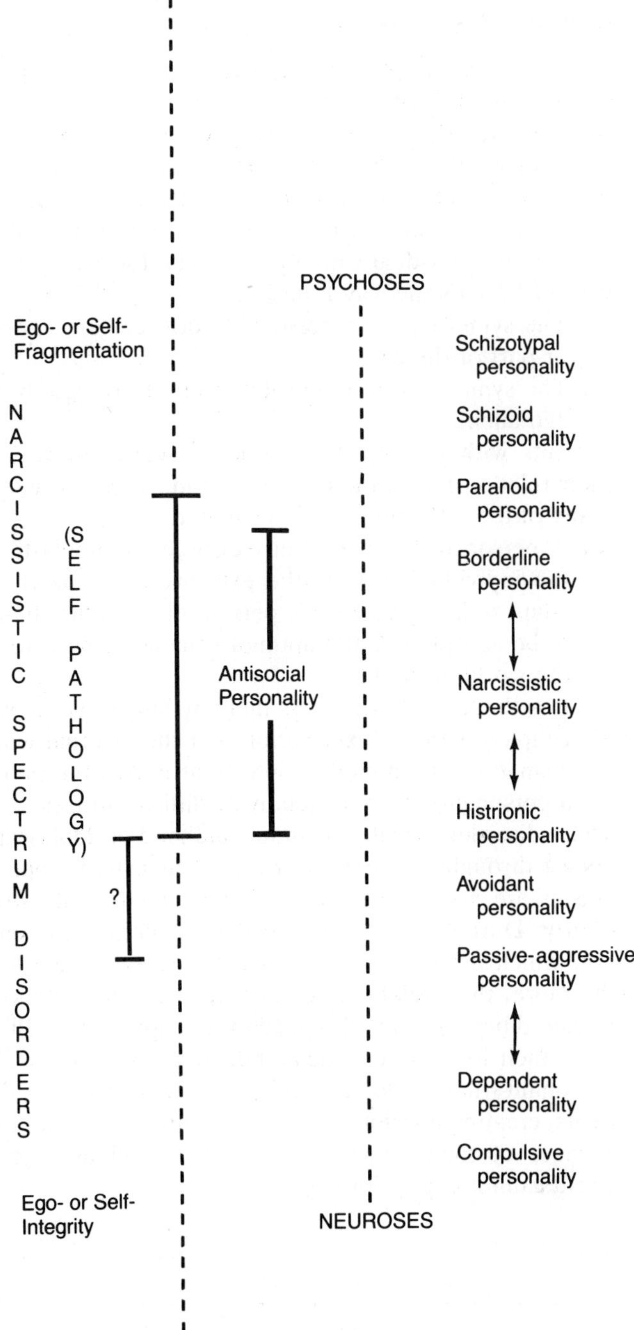

The heavy lines indicate disorders clearly explained as manifestations of self pathology. The dotted lines represent disorders that may possibly be explained as manifestations of self pathology.

Figure 8–1. Personality disorders as related to the theory of self pathology.

C. Clinical Manifestations

A number of characteristics can be identified for all personality disorders, regardless of the specific diagnostic group.

1. The symptoms of a personality disorder are not perceived by the individual as unpleasant. These patients are not usually aware of anything being wrong with them. This is in distinction to the neuroses, in which symptoms are experienced as unpleasant. To an individual with a personality disorder, it is simply a case of "That's the way I am."
   a. The symptoms of a personality disorder are ego-syntonic, or part of the ego.
   b. The symptoms of a neurotic disorder are ego-dystonic, or ego-alien.
2. Patients with personality disorders have a different view of their relationship to the external world, which explains in part many of the difficulties they encounter.
   a. A person with a personality disorder is alloplastic, that is, the individual expects the external world to change and adapt to him. A neurotic person, on the other hand, tends to be autoplastic, attempting to change himself to adapt to the world around him.
   b. It is the lack of awareness that anything is wrong with him, coupled with the expectation that the external world must change to accommodate him, that makes the patient with a personality disorder relatively difficult to treat.
3. These disorders usually begin in childhood or adolescence, and persist throughout adult life. Because their basic coping mechanisms are maladaptive, these individuals tolerate stress very poorly. During periods of stress they experience intense anxiety, which usually resolves when the stress is removed. Furthermore, their relationships and occupational functioning are impaired because of their maladaptive coping skills. In essence, then, their lives are chaotic and disrupted as a result of a basic personality flaw. People usually react negatively to these patients, creating a vicious cycle; they cannot cope with the world because of their personality disorders, and as a result, the world cannot cope with them.

Paranoid Personality

---

a. *Definition:* A personality disorder characterized by a pervasive and unwarranted suspiciousness of others. These individuals have great difficulty trusting others and are hypersensitive to any perceived slight or wrongdoing.

b. Paranoid personalities have a restricted affect. This serves the function of keeping others at a distance, because getting too close intensifies the patient's anxiety and is threatening to him.

c. Associated features:
   - These people are moralistic, with very rigid codes of right and wrong.
   - They often "collect injustices."
   - There is a tendency to misinterpret innocent events as evidence that "everyone is against me." This represents ideas of reference. Paranoid personalities, however, are not grossly delusional or psychotic.
   - Litigiousness is common; these people attempt to "get even" for things done to them, often through the legal system.
   - As would be expected from their distrust of others, the quality of their interpersonal relations is very poor.

Schizoid Personality

a. *Definition:* Schizoid personalities have a defect in the ability to form relationships, as evidenced by a lack of warm, tender feelings, and indifference to praise or criticism. These people come across as withdrawn and aloof, and as preferring solitary activities to the company of others.

b. Schizoid personalities have few, if any, friends and seem to prefer being alone.

c. Their affect can best be described as cold and aloof.

d. The schizoid personality can best be understood as withdrawing from the world of relationships as a way of defending against a fear of rejection. By totally isolating themselves from others, they protect themselves from the pain of rejection and loneliness.

e. Establishing a therapeutic relationship with these patients is extremely difficult.

Schizotypal Personality

a. *Definition:* A personality disorder characterized by oddities of speech, thought, perception, and behavior. These are not severe enough, however, to meet the diagnostic criteria for schizophrenia. They are generally bizarre and eccentric but not psychotic. In addition, these individuals tend to be socially isolated, with poor interpersonal rapport. In this way they share many features in common with the schizoid personality.

b. In the past these patients have sometimes been referred to as simple or latent schizophrenics. It should be emphasized, however, that they are *not* schizophrenic.

c. Associated features:
   - Thought content is marked by autism, magical thinking, bizarre fantasies, and ideas of reference.
   - Illusions, depersonalization, and derealization episodes are common.
   - Affect is most often constricted, but periods of anxiety or depression may occur.
   - Speech is marked by odd or peculiar words, but never reaching psychotic proportions.
   - From the above description, it is easy to imagine how schizotypal personalities may be mistaken for schizophrenia.

Histrionic Personality

a. *Definition:* A personality disorder in which behavior is overly dramatic, reactive, and intensely expressed. These features lead to intense disturbances in interpersonal relationships.

b. Histrionic personalities are lively and dramatic. They tend to exaggerate and often seem to be acting out a role.

c. Their reactions to relatively minor incidents are intense and out of proportion to the actual situations.

d. Although superficially charming, these patients lack genuine warmth and appear shallow.

e. There is a strong tendency for seductive behavior and sexual acting-out.

f. Relationships are unstable and marked by dependency, manipulative behavior, and impulsive suicidal threats or gestures.
g. In the past, this disorder has been called hysterical personality.
h. Although traditionally this disorder has been thought to be more common in women, recent evidence suggests that it is also quite common in men.

Narcissistic Personality

a. *Definition:* Narcissistic personalities are overly preoccupied with themselves. They have a grandiose sense of importance or uniqueness. There is also an exhibitionistic need for attention or praise, often accompanied by a strong sense of entitlement.
b. Relationships are usually unstable and marked by extremes of idealization and devaluation.
c. Underlying the grandiose facade are chronic feelings of emptiness and low self-esteem.
d. Disappointments are reacted to intensely with the expression of narcissistic rage.
e. Others perceive these individuals as cold and lacking empathy, and as only concerned with themselves.
f. Fantasies of power, wealth, beauty, and fame are common.
g. These patients utilize a characteristic defense mechanism called splitting, a primitive defense mechanism in which the patient is unable to internalize both good and bad qualities in the same person. The patient, therefore, perceives significant others as being all good or all bad, with nothing in-between.

Borderline Personality

a. *Definition:* A personality disorder marked by intense instability in a number of areas, including interpersonal relationships, behavior, mood, and self-image.
b. Relationships are intense and unstable. As with the narcissistic personality, extremes of idealization and devaluation may occur.

c. Behavior is frequently impulsive and often self-destructive. Suicidal threats and gestures are common, as are drug and alcohol abuse.
d. Mood is unstable, with rapid shifts from normal to dysphoric. Anger is often intense and inappropriate. Narcissistic rage is commonly seen.
e. Identity disturbances, marked by gender identity confusion and feelings of emptiness and boredom, are often seen. These individuals often need another person to make them feel "whole."
f. Borderline personalities are generally intolerant of being alone and will seek out others to avoid this feeling.
g. Associated features:
   - Frequently perceived as demanding and manipulative.
   - Under stress these patients may experience transient psychotic episodes.
   - They experience almost constant anxiety.
   - Episodes of depersonalization and derealization are common.
   - Splitting is the characteristic defense mechanism, as with narcissistic personalities.
h. Borderline personalities share many features in common with narcissistic, histrionic, antisocial, and schizotypal personalities. Some psychoanalytic theorists view these disorders as part of a narcissistic spectrum, with borderline personality simply representing a more severe variant of the narcissistic personality.

Avoidant Personality

a. *Definition:* A personality disorder in which there is hypersensitivity to potential rejection, shame, or humiliation. As a result, there is reluctance to enter into relationships without guarantees of acceptance or praise. These individuals are withdrawn and have an underlying feeling of low self-esteem.
b. Avoidant personalities differ from schizoid personalities in that the avoidant personality desires relationships but is afraid to enter into them out of fear of rejection. The schizoid patient has no desire for relationships and is more comfortable alone.
c. These individuals often appear helpless and pathetic, at times eliciting the sympathy of others.

d. They lack the coldness and aloofness so often seen in schizoid personalities.

Dependent Personality

a. *Definition:* A personality disorder marked by the tendency to passively allow others to assume control and responsibility for major areas of life. The dependent person subordinates his own needs to those of others, often as a way of gaining acceptance.
b. These people have an intense need to please others.
c. They are unwilling to make demands of others and neglect their own needs and rights. Again, this often occurs out of a fear of rejection.
d. Underlying their dependency is a low self-esteem.

Compulsive Personality

a. *Definition:* A personality disorder in which there is a restricted ability to express emotion, accompanied by a tendency toward perfectionism. These people are overly preoccupied with details and with "doing things right." Because of this, there is a subsequent failure to "grasp the big picture." This disorder is characterized by predominantly anal character traits, as first described by Freud.
b. These people are rigid and preoccupied with rules and regulations.
c. They often appear stingy with both their emotions and their material possessions.
d. Their preoccupation with trivial details often impairs effective functioning.
e. In nonstressful situations they may appear conscientious and productive. Thus, there may be a certain adaptive advantage to this type of personality.
f. Underlying the apparent efficiency, however, is a fear of making mistakes that leads to indecisiveness.

Passive-Aggressive Personality

a. *Definition:* A personality disorder in which there is resistance to demands for adequate performance in both social and occupational functioning. Rather than expressing this resistance directly, however, it is acted out indirectly.

b. These people are usually stubborn and intentionally forgetful, and tend to put off doing what is expected of them.
c. Elements of dependency are commonly present.
d. Most people react angrily to this type of personality.
e. The passive behavior is thought of as a covert expression of aggression, which the person is afraid to express directly.

III. NURSING MANAGEMENT

A. Assessment

1. Does the patient demonstrate any awareness of his problems or does he believe that there is nothing wrong with his behavior?
2. What is the patient's level of anxiety?
3. How does he cope with anxiety and stress? In what manner does he translate anxiety into action?
4. What is the patient's level of frustration tolerance?
5. In what manner does he interact with others?
6. Does he attempt to manipulate staff, family, friends, or other patients? Does he play staff members against one another?
7. Does the patient blame others for all of his problems? Does he blame himself excessively for his problems?
8. Is the patient able to express his feelings? In what manner does he express feelings?
9. Is the patient overly dependent on staff and others?
10. Does the patient continuously demand attention from staff?
11. Does the patient exhibit seductive behavior or sexual acting-out?
12. Does the patient demonstrate attention-seeking behavior (suicide threats, seizure-like activity, or fainting spells)?
13. What is the patient's level of participation in unit activities?
14. Does the patient demonstrate low self-esteem? Very high self-esteem?
15. Does the patient attempt to gain special favors or privileges?
16. Does the patient show sound judgment in making decisions and in setting goals for the future?
17. Is there a history of impulsive behavior (suicide attempts, self-mutilation, or threats and/or harm to others)?
18. Is there a history of substance abuse?
19. What is the patient's legal history?
20. Can the patient control his anger or does he have temper tantrums?

21. What is the quality and number of his interpersonal relationships?
22. Is he able to delay gratification or does he demand immediate satisfaction of his needs and desires?
23. Has the patient gained insight or changed his behavior based on past experience or punishment?
24. How does the patient handle responsibility?
25. Is the patient able to follow rules and obey laws?
26. Can the patient tolerate being alone? Does he seem to require the presence of others?
27. Can the patient tolerate being with others or is he more comfortable alone?
28. How does the patient respond to authority figures? Does he resent and defy authority? Does he overly identify with authority figures?
29. Is he willing to accept treatment?

B. Planning

Planning for the nursing care of the patient with a personality disorder should give consideration to the patient's unique personality traits and needs. For example, the schizoid patient may not be able to tolerate closeness with others and may be less anxious in a private room where he can spend time alone. The dependent patient may fear abandonment and seek constant attention from staff.

Planning should also give consideration to needs of the staff. Patients who demonstrate traits of personality disorders to an excessive degree can create stress for staff who find that patients' responses consistently fall outside the normal range of behavior generally noted in medical-surgical patients.

C. Intervention

1. Prevention

As stated earlier, manifestations of personality disorders can often be recognized during childhood or adolescence. The origin of these disorders can be traced to traumatic relationships with significant figures, usually parents, during the first 3½ years of life. This process was described by Mahler and colleagues (1975) in their stages of separation-individuation. Phase-appropriate, empathic responses by the parents throughout development are the most important factors in preventing the appearance of personality disorders.

Early recognition and treatment of oppositional behavior and conduct disorders may often prevent severe personality pathology from being expressed as an adult. Autistic or overly dependent behavior in children may also signal potential character pathology.

2. Treatment

   Treatment of personality disorders is difficult and long-term. Treatment issues focus on living in the here and now, on careful assessment of thought patterns leading to maladaptive behavior, on the consequences of maladaptive behavior, on establishing new ways of thinking, and on adopting socially acceptable behavior.

3. Medications

   There are no psychotropic medications that address the core pathology in personality disorders. Medication at best provides only symptomatic relief. Antidepressants should be used for those cases in which a superimposed major depression is present. Antipsychotics are useful in those disorders prone to transient psychotic episodes (e.g., borderline and schizotypal personalities). Lithium has been advocated to improve impulse control, but studies have been inconclusive. Benzodiazepines and other anxiolytics should be used with caution because of the potential for abuse and dependence. As a general rule, psychotherapy remains the treatment of choice for the personality disorders.

4. Nursing Actions

   The discussion of nursing actions will be based on both general and specific recommendations for management of patients with personality disorders. As noted previously, Chapter 7 contains a discussion of nursing actions for antisocial personality disorder.

   General Nursing Actions

   a. Provide clear, consistent, and firm expectations based on therapeutic concern for the patient. This helps let the patient know what is expected and provides guidance toward self-control.
   b. Maintain communication and consistency in approach among all members of the treatment team. This will decrease being manipulated and played against one another.
   c. Address, rather than avoid dealing with, the patient and any unacceptable behavior.
   d. Maintain awareness of self and personal attitudes toward the patient in order to avoid being "caught up" in his pathology.
   e. Discuss the consequences of behavior and alternative behaviors with the patient.

f. Focus on the present, the here and now.
g. Hold the patient accountable for his behavior. Threats to harm staff may result in administrative discharge from the hospital. Theft of drugs or other criminal behavior may result in legal action against the patient.
h. Do not discuss personal information about self, other staff members, or other patients.

Nursing Actions for Specific Personality Disorders

a. The Patient with a Paranoid Personality Disorder

   The suspicious patient constantly complains and questions staff about all aspects of his care. He has a tendency to find fault, lacks trust, and may hold real or imagined grudges against the hospital support system.

   - Do not offer reassurances. This will only increase the patient's anxiety and lack of trust.
   - Acknowledge the patient's beliefs without offering opinions about them (e.g., Patient: "I'm not going to take that pill, you're trying to poison me!" Nurse: "Mr. Smith, can you clarify for me what you mean by being poisoned?"). The patient may be experiencing side effects of the medication, he may be suspicious of the staff, or there may be a number of other reasons for his statement. If the patient absolutely refuses to take his medication, the nurse should document this and attempt to give the medication later.
   - Acknowledge the patient's feelings by restating them in words similar to his own (Patient: "All of you doctors and nurses are just using me for a guinea pig!" Nurse: "Having to be in the hospital is frightening for you.").
   - Explain all routines and procedures.
   - Touch the patient only when necessary to give direct care. He cannot tolerate this type of closeness, and his level of anxiety and suspicion may increase.
   - Maintain continuity of daily routine.
   - Enter the patient's room slowly and stand at the foot of the bed or sit when talking with him.
   - Leave the patient with a clear access to the door.

b. The Patient with a Schizoid or Schizotypal Personality Disorder

   This patient may seem aloof and avoid interacting with others. His emotional tone may appear bland or flat. Hospitalization forces him into a proximity with others that may increase his level of anxiety.

   - Place the patient in a private room whenever possible.

- Allow him to spend time alone.
- Avoid touching the patient except when giving direct care.
- Do not probe for emotional responses or deep-seated feelings.
- Keep explanations clear and concise.
- Be aware of the patient's need to maintain physical and emotional distance.

c. The Patient with a Histrionic Personality Disorder

The histrionic patient tends to respond in overly emotional and dramatic ways. He can be captivating and engaging and can induce staff to become overinvolved. This patient may dress and behave seductively and then be surprised when the behavior elicits sexual advances or responses from others.

- Give simple, straightforward, and calm explanations and answers to questions.
- When providing education for this patient, check his comprehension by asking him to repeat the instructions.
- Ask him how he *feels*. Being able to talk about his feelings can reduce stress and anxiety.
- Set firm, consistent, and caring limits for behavior.

d. The Patient with a Narcissistic Personality Disorder

This patient has an exaggerated sense of self-importance. He may expect preferential treatment and insist that the attending physician or chief of staff be his personal physician. He tends to devalue those whom he sees as inferior.

- Restate the patient's statements and feelings back to him in a matter-of-fact, nonjudgmental manner.
- It may be necessary for the nurse manager or head nurse to intervene with the patient on behalf of the staff. The patient's anxiety and need for superiority may decrease when talking with another "authority" figure.
- The above intervention may need repeating in order to give reinforcement and maintain limits that have been set.

e. The Patient with a Borderline Personality Disorder

The borderline patient is often described as immature, inconsistent, and labile. He lacks personal identity and relies on others to make him feel complete. He is prone to impulsive, acting-out behavior to gain attention. Under extreme stress this patient can decompensate into psychosis.

- Be consistent and set firm, clear limits in order to minimize attention-seeking and manipulative behavior.

- Provide a safe environment to protect the patient and others from harm. Place the patient in a room near the nurses' station to facilitate closer observation of the patient. Supervise the patient's use of any sharp or dangerous objects.
- Assist the patient with resolution of any immediate crises.
- Focus on self-responsibility for behavior.

f. The Patient with an Avoidant Personality Disorder

The patient with an avoidant personality disorder is overly sensitive to social stimuli and is hypersensitive to the moods and feelings of others, especially those that could be interpreted as rejection, humiliation, or shame. Although he chooses to isolate himself from closeness with others out of fear of abandonment, he has an extreme need for external structure and control. This patient may be seen by staff as timid, withdrawn, or even cold and strange.

- Present information in a concise, matter-of-fact manner that is less likely to be misinterpreted by the patient.
- Use a calm, nurturing approach.
- Be consistent.
- Avoid making promises that cannot be kept.
- Do not whisper to others in front of the patient. Be cautious about talking or laughing outside of his room, since he is likely to misinterpret these actions.

g. The Patient with a Dependent Personality Disorder

Most patients become somewhat more dependent during hospitalization; however, those patients whose normal personality style is dependent, clingy, needy, and demanding can regress to an extremely dependent level.

- Anticipate the patient's needs to reduce fear of abandonment.
- Set supportive, but firm limits on unrealistic demands.
- When possible, sit and talk with the patient rather than standing. This communicates a sense of interest and caring.
- Terminate patient-staff relationships on discharge from the hospital.

h. The Patient with a Compulsive Personality Disorder

The patient with a compulsive personality disorder appears overly controlled and orderly. He tends to think or intellectualize rather than feel. Ambiguity and anticipation of loss can provoke extreme anxiety in this patient.

- Provide careful and thorough explanations of procedures, medications, and tests.

- Answer all questions patiently and respectfully. This patient needs to know what is happening and the reasons in order to feel in control.
- Allow the patient to set bath schedules, medication schedules, and other aspects of care whenever possible. The ability to make choices can enhance the patient's sense of control.

i. The Patient with a Passive-Aggressive Personality Disorder

The passive-aggressive patient is unable to express anger directly toward another individual; therefore, he expresses his anger indirectly in ways that are often self-defeating and in some way offensive to the other person. Examples of passive-aggressive behavior include "pouting, procrastination, stubbornness, and intentional inefficiency" (Schultz and Dark 1986).

- Set clear, firm, consistent limits. Do not justify, argue, or bargain with the patient about the limits.
- Maintain frequent staff communication in order to decrease manipulation.
- Enforce hospital policies, rules, and regulations in a consistent, firm manner.

D. Evaluation/Expected Outcomes

1. The nurse will:
   a. Explain rules, regulations, and limits in a clear, firm, yet caring manner.
   b. Set and enforce limits in a consistent, therapeutic manner.
   c. Communicate frequently with other staff members to facilitate consistency and to decrease the patient's manipulative and attention-seeking behavior.
2. The patient will:
   a. Identify behaviors and other considerations that led to hospitalization.
   b. Avoid harm to himself or others.
   c. Function within the limits and regulations of the environment.
   d. Demonstrate socially acceptable ways to deal with frustration and anger.
   e. Increase impulse control and eliminate acting-out behavior such as temper tantrums, suicide threats, and promiscuity.

E. Evaluation for Referral

The patient with a personality disorder may be admitted to a medical-surgical unit because of a suicide attempt (e.g., overdose, wrist-slashing, or gunshot wound), an unexpected accident, or a physical illness. Any patient who is suicidal or homicidal should be placed on a closed psychiatric unit as soon as the medical-surgical condition permits. The psychiatric nurse clinical specialist or psychiatric liaison nurse can be consulted to assist with planning care and setting limits while the patient is on a medical-surgical unit. Referral for psychiatric treatment after hospitalization should be offered, but frequently this patient will see no need for psychiatric care, believing that there is nothing wrong with him.

IV. POTENTIAL NURSING DIAGNOSES

1. Adjustment, impaired, related to
   - lack of insight
   - dependency needs
   - inadequate skills for management of daily living
   - changes or crises
2. Anxiety, related to
   - feelings of inadequacy, worthlessness, or hopelessness
   - dependency needs
   - history of limited success
   - fear
3. Coping, ineffective individual, related to
   - poor social skills
   - hostility or anger
   - poor impulse control
   - dependency needs
   - impaired judgment
4. Noncompliance, related to
   - disregard for the needs of others
   - inability to delay gratification
   - feelings of entitlement
5. Self-concept, disturbance in, related to
   - history of limited success
   - dependency needs
   - low self-esteem
6. Self-harm, potential for, related to
   - poor impulse control
   - manipulative behavior
   - impaired judgment
   - poor self-esteem

7. Sexuality patterns, altered, related to
   - disturbance in perceptions of self
   - dependency needs
   - manipulative behavior
   - disregard for acceptable social behavior
   - disregard for needs of others
8. Social interaction, impaired, related to
   - disregard for rights and feelings of others
   - failure to learn from past experiences
   - feelings of entitlement
9. Violence, potential for, related to
   - poor impulse control
   - disregard for socially acceptable behavior
   - anger, hostility
   - lack of feelings of remorse
   - inability to delay gratification

V. SUMMARY

The personality disorders are characterized by long-standing patterns of maladaptive behavior that cause significant impairment in social and occupational functioning. Although a number of distinct personality disorders can be identified, often patients present with mixed features of several different types of personality disorders. At times, particularly during periods of severe stress, individuals with healthy personalities will regress and temporarily display signs of character pathology. When the stress resolves, these pathological traits will disappear.

Patients with personality disorders tolerate stress and frustration poorly. They are prone to periods of anxiety and depression, with depression often being the presenting feature. These patients often overreact to medical or surgical illnesses, displaying regressed, dependent behavior or reacting in a hostile, demanding manner. If these behaviors are not understood as manifestations of an underlying personality disorder, negative staff reactions are likely to ensue.

The treatment of choice for personality disorders is long-term psychotherapy, most often combining both supportive and insight-oriented approaches. Medication, particularly antidepressants and low-dose antipsychotic agents, may be useful adjuncts to treatment, but should not be the primary treatment modality utilized.

While often difficult to treat, this group of disorders provides a fascinating glimpse of psychopathology. Contemporary psychoanalytic theorists, such as Kohut and Kernberg, have outlined complicated dynamic theories that have increased our understanding of personality development, both normal and abnormal. Although a great deal has been learned about the personality disorders, much remains to be uncovered.

References

American Psychiatric Association (1980). *Diagnostic and statistical manual of mental disorders* (3rd ed.). Washington, DC: American Psychiatric Association.

American Psychiatric Association (1987). *Diagnostic and statistical manual of mental disorders* (3rd ed.). Washington, DC: American Psychiatric Association.

Barry, P. D. (1984). *Psychological nursing assessment and intervention.* Philadelphia: J. B. Lippincott Company.

Frosch, J. P. (1983). The treatment of antisocial and borderline personality disorders. *Hospital and community psychiatry, 34*(3), 243–248.

Gunderson, J. G. (1984). *Borderline personality disorder.* Washington, DC: American Psychiatric Press.

Kernberg, O. (1975). *Borderline conditions and pathological narcissism.* New York: Aronson.

Kernberg, O. (1984). *Severe personality disorders.* New Haven: Yale University Press.

Kohut, H. (1971). *The analysis of the self.* New York: International Universities Press.

Kohut, H., and Wolfe, E. (1978). The disorders of the self and their treatment: An outline. *International Journal of Psychoanalysis, 59,* 413–425.

Mahler, M. S., Pine, F., and Bergman, A. (1975). *The psychological birth of the human infant.* New York: Basic Books.

McLane, A. M. (Ed.) (1987). *Classification of nursing diagnoses,* Proceedings of the Seventh Conference—North American Nursing Diagnosis Association. St. Louis: C. V. Mosby Company.

Masterson, J. F. (1981). *The narcissistic and borderline disorders: An integrated developmental approach.* New York: Brunner/Mazel.

Platt-Koch, L. M. (1983). Borderline personality disorder—A therapeutic approach. *American Journal of Nursing, 83*(12), 1666–1671.

Schultz, J. M., and Dark, S. L. (1986). *Manual of psychiatric nursing care plans* (2nd ed.). Boston: Little, Brown & Company.

SECTION THREE

ADDICTIVE BEHAVIORS AND CHEMICAL DEPENDENCY

Chapter 9

The Patient with an Eating Disorder: Anorexia Nervosa and Bulimia

Nancy D. Stephens *Roberta L. Messner*

I. STATEMENT OF PURPOSE

Eating disorders, characterized by gross disturbances in eating behaviors, have reached nearly epidemic proportions in the Western world over the last decade. Although anorexia nervosa, bulimia, pica, rumination disorder of infancy, and atypical eating disorder are all included under the broad category of "eating disorders," this chapter will address only the two most common: anorexia nervosa and bulimia.

While anorexia nervosa and bulimia (without weight loss) are separate syndromes, they are manifestations of closely related underlying emotional symptoms. These disorders are closely tied to personality styles and disorders. They are immensely destructive to the physical and emotional health of the patient and the family unit. Failure to recognize the psychosocial and physical symptoms early in the course of these disorders can result in long-term physical and emotional problems and/or death.

Because the majority of individuals with anorexia nervosa and bulimia are female, the patient will be referred to as "she."

II. OVERVIEW OF EATING DISORDERS

Anorexia Nervosa

A. Description of the Illness

Anorexia nervosa is a psychological disorder manifested by voluntary self-inflicted starvation. Untreated, the syndrome may lead to death. The disorder centers on the patient's need to establish a sense of control and identity. The patient characteristically perceives her emaciated body as "fat," denies the illness, and is resistant to treatment.

Approximately 50% of anorectics, however, are unable to continue self-starvation and succumb to eating binges followed by self-induced vomiting (Burckes 1983). Only 55% of anorectics develop strong personal relationships or marry. Forty-eight percent of anorectics reside with parents, and 90% are employed (Burckes 1983).

Anorexia nervosa was first described in 1689 by Richard Morton, with the classic symptoms of appetite loss, extreme wasting without lassitude, and amenorrhea in females (Hay and Leonard 1979). The cause of anorexia nervosa is still unknown, but it has been associated with a hypothalamic disorder and possible endocrine and neurophysiological factors. Also implicated is a distorted self-image in which the individual inaccurately perceives her emaciated body as grotesquely overweight.

The course of anorexia continues until death in 15–21% of cases (American Psychiatric Association 1987). Researchers estimate that among anorectics that are treated, 49% will restore weight, 31% will exhibit weight fluctuations or become obese, and 18% will remain anorectic (Burckes, 1983).

B. Incidence

It is estimated that one out of every 100,000 people will develop anorexia nervosa each year, yet the illness seems to predominate in Western white females, among whom the incidence may be as high as one in 200. A dramatic increase in the syndrome has been noted in the last ten years, and a report from Zimbabwe may indicate an unknown incidence in third-world countries (Zucker 1984). While the diagnosis in males is hampered by the lack of one classic symptom—menstrual disorders—and by the lack of awareness of its occurrence, reports from sports medicine programs are revealing a greater incidence of anorexia nervosa in males than has been thought (Zucker 1984).

Surveys indicate that the syndrome is prevalent in all economic sectors of our society and indeed may prevail in all upwardly mobile industrial societies, contradicting previous reports that anorexia is primarily a problem existing in upper-class populations in the West. Anorexia nervosa has been found to be more prevalent among sisters and mothers of patients with the syndrome than in the general population (American Psychiatric Association 1987) and more common in families where there is a sibling with a chronic illness or a learning disability (Zucker 1984).

C. Clinical Manifestations

Clinical manifestations of anorexia nervosa may include the following:

1. Emaciation with loss of subcutaneous fat and loss of normal body contours
2. Distorted body image—patient perceives her emaciated body as "fat"
3. Cessation of menstrual periods, which often occurs before noticeable weight loss
4. Weight loss of 25% body weight with no known physical illness that would account for the loss
5. Incapacitating sense of ineffectiveness
6. Hyperactivity
7. Food binges followed by fasting, vomiting, and/or overuse of laxatives
8. Depression
9. Constipation
10. Dependent edema
11. Loss of scalp hair
12. Lanugo, or growth of fine body hair, which is thought to be a primitive response to help conserve body heat
13. Intolerance of cold temperatures
14. Bradycardia
15. Electrolyte imbalance from binging or purging
16. Inaccurate perception of hunger and other body sensations (i.e., fatigue as manifested by hyperactivity)
17. Hypotension, including postural hypotension
18. Alkalosis
19. Elevated blood urea
20. Suicidal ideation (approximately 25% of patients attempt suicide) (Sanger and Cassino 1984)
21. Bizarre or ritualistic behavior
22. Preoccupation with food, body image, and becoming obese
23. Manipulative behavior
24. May be very knowledgeable about nutrition
25. Disproportionate decrease in high-carbohydrate and high-fat foods
26. Abuse of laxatives and diuretics
27. Dry, scaly skin with yellow carotenemic hue, along with elevated serum carotene levels
28. Mild anemia
29. Decreased white blood count
30. Diminished libido in adults
31. Stunted psychosexual development

32. Petechiae
33. Loss of bone density
34. Prolonged QT intervals on electrocardiogram, indicating susceptibility to life-threatening cardiac arrhythmias
35. Decrease in body temperature by approximately 1°C
36. Pimples and fine rash

Bulimia

A. Description of the Illness

The syndrome of bulimia was first observed around 1940 in connection with anorexia nervosa. Bulimia was officially designated as a disorder distinct from anorexia nervosa by the American Psychiatric Association in 1980.

Bulimia is an episodic eating disorder of unknown cause that involves alternating binges and purges. A "binge" is the rapid ingestion of large amounts of high-caloric foods. When the individual feels physically uncomfortable due to gastric distention, she feels remorseful and attempts to "purge" her body of ingested food by self-induced vomiting, use of cathartics or diuretics, or rigorous dieting or fasting. While the anorectic is morbidly obsessed with thinness, the bulimic is morbidly obsessed with fatness (Burckes 1983). The bulimic seems to use food as a temporary relief in stressful situations.

Bulimia is often incapacitating in those individuals who constantly "binge" or "purge." However, while the disorder appears to be chronic and intermittent over many years, studies indicate that less than 50% of bulimics seek professional help. Deceptive periods of normal eating patterns or of normal eating patterns and fasts may alternate with periods of bulimia.

B. Incidence

Like anorexia, bulimia appears to be present in all economic sectors of our society. The disorder is predominant in females (American Psychiatric Association 1987), although 20% are male (Burckes 1983). However, it seems to be more widespread than anorexia nervosa, with an estimated 500,000–1,000,000 bulimics in the United States alone (Burckes 1983). As many as 15% to 20% of American college women binge and purge as a means of inhibiting weight gain (Zucker 1984). Little is available on familial patterns except that obesity is frequently present in parents or siblings. It is difficult to assess the true scope of this disorder, since bulimics tend to be very secretive and most cases are never reported.

C. Clinical Manifestations

Clinical manifestations of bulimia may include the following:

1. Recurrent episodes of inconspicuous (closet) binge eating, ranging from 1,000 to greater than 50,000 calories per binge. The average binge is 3000–5000 calories (Burckes 1983)
2. Termination of a binge due to abdominal pain, social interruption, or self-induced vomiting
3. Frequent weight fluctuation of greater than 10 pounds (American Psychiatric Association 1987)
4. Awareness that eating behavior is abnormal, accompanied by a fear of not being able to stop eating voluntarily
5. Feelings of depression and guilt after a binge
6. More normal appearance than the anorectic, with weight generally within normal range (American Psychiatric Association 1987)
7. Intermittent substance abuse, most frequently barbiturates, amphetamines, or alcohol (American Psychiatric Association 1987)
8. Menstrual irregularities
9. Enlargement of parotid gland due to acidic vomitus
10. Poor impulse control
11. Low self-esteem
12. Suicidal ideation or overt suicidal attempts (approximately 23% of patients attempt suicide) (Garfinkel et al. 1980)
13. Urinary tract infections
14. Electrolyte imbalance from binging and purging
15. Seizures
16. Erosion of tooth enamel or gingivitis from acidic vomitus
17. Chronic irritation of the mouth; chronic sore throat
18. Puffiness around eyes, broken blood vessels on face, or scars on fingers, due to trauma from self-induced vomiting
19. Compulsive stealing, both of food and money to purchase food; as much as $50–$100 a day can be spent for food (Burckes 1983)
20. Chronic hoarseness
21. Abuse of laxatives and diuretics.

III. NURSING MANAGEMENT

A. Assessment

Assessment of the patient with anorexia nervosa or bulimia involves a comprehensive physical and psychosocial nursing appraisal. Because these two disorders are closely related, the following assessment criteria can be adapted to either clinical situation:

1. Assess potential for self-harm:
   a. Assess feelings of depression, guilt, and ineffectiveness
   b. Suicidal ideation
   c. Verbalization of self-deprecating thoughts
2. Assess nutritional status:
   a. Height/weight
   b. Percentage of weight loss or fluctuations in weight
   c. Rule out any known physical illness to account for weight loss
   d. Biochemical laboratory values, particularly serum albumin, total protein, total lymphocyte count, total iron-binding capacity, and serum transfer, to assess visceral protein status and to establish baseline levels prior to refeeding
   e. Anthropometric measurements to determine muscle mass and fat reserves
   f. Delayed hypersensitivity tests to assess immunocompetence
   g. Dietary habits/eating patterns may be highly variable (e.g., self-starvation, repeated fad dieting, binge eating, purging through self-induced vomiting, and use of laxatives or diuretics)
3. Assess clinical data to determine if starvation is approaching:
   a. Fluid and electrolyte imbalance
   b. Cardiac arrhythmias (may indicate an electrolyte imbalance or a wasting myocardium)
   c. Presence of ketone bodies in the urine
   d. Presence of infection (may indicate diminished immune status)
4. Assess additional pertinent laboratory values for abnormalities:
   a. Electrolytes
   b. Thyroid levels
   c. Complete blood count with differential white blood count
5. Assess level of mental acuity (e.g., ability to concentrate).
6. Assess menstrual pattern (e.g., erratic cycle or amenorrhea).
7. Assess body image (e.g., disturbances in or delusions regarding body proportions).
8. Assess cognitive interpretation of stimuli (e.g., inaccurate awareness of hunger or fatigue).
9. Assess exercise patterns (extensive calisthenics or other exercise; sleep deprivation; use of stimulants).
10. Assess other physical manifestations for each disorder (refer to the "Clinical Manifestations" listed previously for anorexia nervosa and bulimia).

B. Planning

Planning of the nursing care for the patient with anorexia nervosa or bulimia should be founded on a comprehensive nursing assessment and the formation of nursing diagnoses. Modification of the nursing care plan should be based on ongoing reassessments of the patient's physical and psychosocial status and evaluation of the nursing interventions.

C. Intervention

1. Prevention

The nurse possesses the knowledge base so important for prompt recognition of early warning signs and symptoms of eating disorders. Poor prognosis is associated with the existence of active disease for longer than two years and greater than 25% weight loss (Zucker 1984). During the developmental phases of eating disorders, the behaviors of patients are often less rigid and therefore more responsive to therapy. Timely professional intervention is imperative to prevent irreversible or life-threatening consequences.

Early warning clues in the preanorectic patient may include:

a. Altered perception of body size, disturbance in body image, or intense fear of becoming obese
b. Misinterpretation of external and internal stimuli (e.g., perception of hunger)
c. Overwhelming sense of ineffectiveness and powerlessness
d. Dieting to extremes accompanied by an obsession with shopping for and preparation of food (e.g., food rituals, cutting or rearranging food)
e. Adherence to rigid attitudes and compulsive, overly compliant, perfectionistic behavior
f. Social isolation, withdrawal, or depression
g. Regression
h. Disturbances in sleep patterns
i. Hyperactivity
j. Impaired personal identity
k. History of childhood obesity

Early warning signs in the prebulimic patient are less well defined. Bulimia is often a counterpart of anorexia nervosa. Early detection of bulimia is further inhibited by the absence of overt symptoms and the secrecy of the disorder. The bulimic may appear to be the ideal career woman, student, and/or married woman, but beneath this veneer she is acutely disturbed and acknowledges her abnormal eating patterns. However, the bulimic tends to be more concerned with eating and its control, while the anorectic is more preoccupied with weight.

Parents may neglect the compliant, bright, preanorectic child, focusing all efforts on the "problem child" in the family. Nurses can be alert for the aforementioned symptoms to help family members, other health care providers, and the community at large to identify early warning signs of eating disorders. Nurses have many unique opportunities for early case finding through screening programs, outpatient clinics, and community health centers, and can exert a major role in leadership and collaborative activities.

2. Treatment

While the specific treatments of choice in eating disorders remain controversial, early treatment is imperative, since once behavioral and eating patterns have been established, they are notoriously difficult to change. The patient may be highly resistant to treatment initially. Ideally, a clinician of average weight should care for these patients. Treatment consists of a combination of medical, nutritional, and psychiatric therapy.

a. Anorexia Nervosa

The goals of treatment for the anorectic patient include:

- Correction of malnutrition and restoration of normal nutrition
- Resolution of underlying psychological problems
- Development of more appropriate attitudes toward food
- Utilization of more effective coping strategies to address the underlying conflicts
- Correction of disturbed patterns of family interaction

When these goals cannot be met on an outpatient basis, hospitalization is necessary, as indicated in the following situations (Carino and Chmelko 1983):

- Loss of 25% or more body weight
- Threat of serious electrolyte imbalance
- Severe depression with suicidal ideation
- Intensive familial conflicts
- Noncompliance with outpatient treatment regimen

b. Bulimia

Bulimia is often treated on an outpatient basis. The goals of treatment include:

- Interruption of the binge/purge cycle by assisting the patient to gain control of eating (Purging represents both a physical and psychological undoing of binging.)

- Improvement of patient's attitudes toward food, eating, body size, and self

Nutritional Intervention

A comprehensive discussion of nutritional modalities is beyond the scope of this chapter. The nurse is referred to the clinical dietitian and/or nutritional support team for specific information.

In life-threatening situations, aggressive nutritional intervention assumes paramount importance. Nutritional rehabilitation is an important prerequisite to psychosocial rehabilitation as well. Keep in mind that patients with these disorders may attempt to interrupt or sabotage delivery of parenteral or enteral feedings, often leading to life-threatening complications. Such behavior may even represent a suicide attempt. It should be stressed to the patient that nutritional support is not a punitive measure. A variety of enteral or parenteral nutritional measures may be employed, dependent on the particular situation. Refer to hospital policies and procedures for specific information on the administration of enteral or parenteral nutrition. Because edema may occur as a normal part of the refeeding process, the patient should be reassured in a calm, supportive manner that she is not becoming fat and that fluid retention is due to a temporary shift in body fluids.

Enteral Nutrition

Enteral nutrition, the preferred method of nutrient delivery, can be accomplished by the ingestion of a standard diet or by the infusion of a nutritionally complete liquid formula delivered by means of a feeding tube. Feeding tubes are generally of the nasogastric/nasoenteric or gastrostomy/jejunostomy type. The preferred nasogastric/nasoenteric feeding tube should be of small bore and pliable to facilitate patient comfort and decrease the likelihood of mucosal erosion. The tip of the enteral tube can be placed in the stomach (nasogastric), the duodenum (nasoduodenal), or the jejunum (nasojejunal). The latter two sites render attempts at self-induced vomiting more difficult.

In the anorectic patient it should be remembered that the highly visible nasogastric/nasoenteric feeding tube may further distort the patient's already misperceived self-image. In such a situation, a gastrostomy/jejunostomy tube may be preferred, as they are less visible and therefore may be less stigmatizing and better accepted. A percutaneous endoscopic gastrostomy (PEG) feeding catheter or a percutaneous endoscopic jejunostomy (PEJ) feeding catheter inserted via gastrointestinal endoscopy may be excellent choices for these patients.

Enteral formula may be administered by three methods:

a. Bolus of a specific amount of formula (usually 200–300 cc) according to a specific schedule (usually every 24 hours)
b. Continuous or intermittent gravity drip
c. Continuous to intermittent infusion via enteral feeding pump

Patients receiving enteral nutrition via tube should be monitored for:

a. Routine lab values
b. Fluid balance: intake and output
c. Weight
d. Formula tolerance (gastrointestinal discomfort, diarrhea)
e. Complications such as retention of feedings or pulmonary aspiration
f. Proper tube placement

Central Parenteral Nutrition

Central parenteral nutrition (CPN) carries a higher risk of infectious, metabolic, mechanical, and technical complications than enteral nutrition. However, it is life-saving when the gastrointestinal tract is either unavailable or unable to tolerate the large amounts of nutrients the anorectic patient may require. CPN consists of a special intravenous solution of amino acids and dextrose. It is administered via a large, central vein (e.g., subclavian, internal or external jugular, or femoral). The subclavian vein is associated with the lowest risk of infection.

A tunneled, right atrial catheter with a Dacron cuff (e.g., the Hickman or Groshong catheter) implanted surgically may be used for long-term nutritional support. This type of catheter is more difficult for the patient to remove and is associated with fewer infectious complications.

CPN is always administered by means of a special intravenous infusion pump. Patients receiving CPN should be monitored for:

a. In-depth laboratory values
b. Fluid balance: intake and output
c. Weight
d. Symptoms of infection
e. Catheter dislodgment
f. Tubing disconnection
g. Air embolism
h. Equipment malfunction

3. Psychotherapeutic Interventions

   A variety, and often a combination, of psychotherapeutic approaches may be utilized in the treatment of eating disorders. Because malnutrition impairs the patient's capacity for rational thinking and behavior, a certain level of nutritional restoration is necessary prior to psychotherapy. Four major therapy approaches are as follows:

   a. Individual Psychotherapy—This one to one approach focuses on resolution of basic conflicts manifested in eating disorders (i.e., issues of low self-image, control, fear of weight gain, guilt, and anxiety).
   b. Family Therapy—This approach recognizes that eating disorders are a family-oriented problem and that family dynamics play a major role in the development and maintenance of eating disorders. Family communication, anxiety, and conflicts are explored with the goal of achieving a stronger, more functional family system.
   c. Behavior Modification—This treatment may be used to modify thoughts and feelings associated with food by rewarding normal eating and discouraging self-induced starvation, binging, and purging.
   d. Group Therapy—This approach ranges from a structured, professionally led setting to self-help lay groups. Group therapy can provide a safe, supportive forum for sharing thoughts and feelings, perceptions of self, and for practicing newly learned behavior. Group therapy seems to be the most effective initial approach in changing bulimic behavior.

      Relaxation exercises, guided imagery, biofeedback, neurolinguistic programming, and assertiveness training may be helpful for patients who are capable of utilizing self-help methods. Rapport, trust, and knowledge of eating disorders are more important criteria for therapists than a particular school of thought. The length of therapy ranges from several sessions to several years. Many experts contend that eating disorders are never cured, but only arrested. Because relapses are common in eating disorders, long-term therapy is indicated.

4. Medications

   Antidepressants, such as tricyclics and monoamine oxidase (MAO) inhibitors, are the primary pharmacological agents used as an adjunct to psychotherapy. MAO inhibitors require specific dietary restrictions (e.g., elimination of foods that contain the amino acid tyramine, such as cheddar and strong or aged cheese, chocolate, yogurt, and some wines). Amphetamines and various other medications taken in combination with MAO inhibitors can also prove dangerous. Antianxiety agents may be useful in selected cases. Antidepressant medications appear to be more promising in the treatment of bulimia than anorexia nervosa. Dilantin (phenytoin sodium) has been helpful in the treatment of some cases of binge eating.

Patients should be carefully monitored for drug levels and possible side effects. There is concern that some patients with eating disorders cannot control their impulses enough to take prescribed medication. In addition, since some of these patients have addictive personalities, they may abuse the medications.

5. Nursing Actions

Nursing care of the patient with an eating disorder is based on physiological, psychosocial, and cultural factors. Specific nursing interventions are as follows:

a. Initiate appropriate precautions to protect the patient from self-harm (e.g., self-induced starvation, suicidal behavior, complications from manipulation of enteral or parenteral nutritional support, injury resulting from diminished sensitivity to temperature and pain, or exhaustion from hyperactivity).
b. Assess for physical/physiological consequences of self-starvation, binging, and purging (i.e., malnutrition, electrolyte imbalance, or infection).
c. Institute appropriate nutritional measures (enteral or parenteral) to correct malnutrition and maintain ideal body weight.
d. Assess the patient's nutritional status to determine ideal body weight and to establish nutritional goals for evaluation of progress.
e. If the patient is able to take oral feedings, foster adequate dietary intake. Initially give a 1500-calorie diet. After one week, progress to a 3000-5000-calorie diet (Howe et al. 1984). Record food/fluid intake. (The patient's obsessive-compulsive behavior may be positively utilized by having her keep a food diary.)
f. Provide a calm, nonthreatening atmosphere with structured observation and support during and 30 minutes after mealtime to lessen the likelihood of binge/purge cycle.
g. Prevent and observe for infectious, metabolic, mechanical, or technical complications of nutrition support therapy.
h. Establish a supportive, trusting therapeutic relationship with the patient and family to facilitate the building of self-esteem and acceptance.

i. Assist in the clarification of patient/family communication patterns.
j. Provide positive reinforcement as weight gain is achieved.
k. Help the patient terminate the abuse of purgatives.
l. Suggest dietary fiber or psyllium supplement, glycerin suppositories, and physical exercise within moderation to re-establish normal peristalsis after chronic laxative abuse.
m. After the appropriate level of nutritional restoration is achieved, explore with the patient feelings of poor self-esteem, ineffectiveness, loss of control, self-awareness, sexuality, and the meaning of food and eating patterns.
n. Recommend that patient engage in distracting activity when she feels the urge to binge.
o. Initiate staff conferences for multidisciplinary planning and collaboration.
p. Refer the patient and family to mental health professionals with expertise in the treatment of eating disorders and to other supportive networks, to assist in the understanding and resolving of underlying psychological conflicts.
q. Initiate referral to a clinical dietitian or nutrition support team for in-depth nutritional assessment and counseling.

D. Evaluation/Expected Outcomes

Measurement of treatment outcomes should be based on physical, psychosocial, cultural, and economic factors. In both anorexia nervosa and bulimia, weight gain and maintenance alone are unreliable indicators of progress, since relapses are common. Nursing intervention will be evaluated by the following criteria, keeping in mind that a significant period of time may elapse before all of these criteria are met.

1. The nurse will:
   a. Foster adequate nutritional intake to achieve and/or maintain ideal body weight.
   b. Explore feelings of self-esteem, guilt, anger, and depression with the patient, assisting her in formation of a realistic body image.
   c. Provide psychological support, helping the patient to change her attitudes toward self and food, and to develop alternative methods of coping with life.
2. The patient will:
   a. Demonstrate the expected responses to nutritional intervention by stabilizing weight initially, gaining ½–2 lbs/wk until ideal body weight is attained, and then maintaining ideal body weight.

b. Utilize measures of nutritional support that will maintain or improve nutritional status.
c. Experience no preventable infectious, metabolic, technical, or mechanical complications from nutritional support modalities and/or nursing intervention.
d. Demonstrate adequate knowledge of the nutritional requirements and of measures to achieve them.
e. Achieve control over eating and life.
f. Gain insight into the urge to engage in self-starvation, uncontrollable binge eating, self-induced vomiting, or excessive use of diuretics, laxatives, and enemas, and cease such activities.
g. Achieve restitution of menstrual cycle.
h. Realize a satisfactory occupational and sexual adjustment.
i. Verbalize positive feelings about self and avoid activities that foster social isolation.

E. Evaluation for Referral

Patients with eating disorders present a very complicated clinical picture and are difficult to treat. They should be referred for treatment to private or community psychiatric/psychological practitioners with expertise in treatment of eating disorders.

IV. POTENTIAL NURSING DIAGNOSES (Kim et al. 1984)

1. Anxiety (mild, moderate, severe), related to
   - guilt or anger
   - low self-esteem
   - feelings of worthlessness and hopelessness
2. Body image disturbance, related to
   - delusions
   - fear of obesity
   - low self-esteem
   - distorted perceptions of reality
3. Bowel elimination, alteration in, related to
   - laxative use or abuse
   - inadequate dietary intake
   - inappropriate eating patterns
4. Communication, impaired, related to
   - feelings of inadequacy
   - secretive behavior
   - social isolation

5. Conflict, decisional: unresolved independence-dependence, related to
   - impaired judgment
   - distortion of reality
   - low self-esteem
6. Coping, ineffective individual/family, related to
   - poor interpersonal skills
   - distortion of reality
7. Family process, alteration in, related in
   - inappropriate, manipulative, and/or secretive behavior
   - poor communication skills
8. Fear, related to
   - distortion of reality
   - feelings of helplessness and powerlessness
9. Fluid volume deficit, related to
   - abnormal fluid loss
   - inadequate dietary intake
   - vomiting
   - use or abuse of laxatives and diuretics
10. Health maintenance, alteration in, related to
    - malnutrition
    - neglect of appropriate health requirements
11. Injury, potential for, related to
    - suicidal ideation
    - malnutrition
    - low self-esteem
    - lowered mental acuity
    - inability to adequately perceive and respond to environmental hazards
12. Knowledge deficit, related to
    - denial
    - impaired thought processes
13. Noncompliance, related to
    - denial
    - delusions
    - intense fear of obesity
14. Nutrition, alterations in: less than body requirements, related to inadequate dietary intake
    - vomiting
    - use and abuse of laxatives
15. Oral mucous membrane, alteration in, related to
    - fluid depletion
    - self-induced vomiting
    - poor hygiene

16. Parenting, alteration in, related to dysfunctional family system
17. Self-care deficit, related to
    - altered thought processes
    - poor hygiene
18. Self-concept, disturbance in, related to
    - body image
    - self-esteem
    - role performance
    - personal identity
19. Sensory-perceptual alteration, related to
    - impaired mental acuity
    - disturbances in thought process
20. Sexual dysfunction, related to
    - decreased interest
    - impaired physical functioning
    - regression
21. Skin integrity, impairment of, related to
    - malnutrition
    - poor hygiene
22. Sleep pattern disturbances, related to
    - compulsive behavior
    - malnutrition
    - hyperactivity
    - depression
23. Social isolation, related to
    - poor self-esteem
    - regression
    - anger
    - feelings of inadequacy
    - impaired social skills
24. Spiritual distress (distress of the human spirit), related to
    - delusions
    - depression
    - feelings of inadequacy and worthlessness
25. Thought processes, alteration in, related to
    - delusions
    - malnutrition
    - regression
    - impaired perception

V. SUMMARY

The problem of eating disorders is widespread, permeating all levels of society in virtually epidemic proportions. External societal influences contribute greatly to the development of eating disorders. Because of the conflicting pressures of today's world and our society's relentless promotion of beauty and success, there is little doubt that the incidence of eating disorders will continue to accelerate.

It is estimated that there are millions of victims of anorexia nervosa and bulimia in the United States alone. Often a secret agony, eating disorders are symbolic of a desperate attempt to cope with life. The patient's real problems are hidden further, however, by a relentless, oppressive pursuit of thinness and weight control.

Anorexia nervosa and bulimia are extremely complex disorders in which the physiological, psychosocial, familial, and cultural aspects are so integrated that it is impossible to treat one without treating the others.

The effects of eating disorders are not only physiologically and psychosocially catastrophic, but have financial and legal ramifications as well. The widespread effects of eating disorders may well reach crisis proportions in this decade.

While the prevention and treatment of eating disorders are both challenging and compelling, the grim outlook can be brighter if symptoms are recognized early and intervention is timely and appropriate. This represents a profound, multidisciplinary responsibility.

References

American Psychiatric Association. (1987). *Diagnostic and statistical manual of mental disorders (DSM III-R).* Washington, DC: American Psychiatric Association.

Bruch, H. (1973). *Eating disorders: Obesity, anorexia nervosa and the person within.* New York: Basic Books, Inc.

Burckes, M. E. (1983). Eating disorders. *The Journal of Practical Nursing* (July/August); 20–24.

Carino, C. M., and Chmelko, P. (1983). Disorders of eating in adolescence: Anorexia and bulimia. *Nursing Clinics of North America, 18*(2), 343–352.

Casper, R. C. (1983). On the emergence of bulimia nervosa as a syndrome—A historical view. *International Journal of Eating Disorders, 2*(3), 2–16.

Cauwels, J. (1983). *Bulimia.* Garden City, NY: Doubleday & Co.

Drossman, D. A., Ontjes, D., and Heizer, W. D. (1979). Anorexia nervosa. *Gastroenterology, 77,* 1115.

Garfinkel, P. E., et al. (1980). The heterogeneity of anorexia nervosa: Bulimia as a distinct subgroup. *Arch. Gen. Psychiatry, 37*(g), 1036–1040.

Hay, G. G., and Leonard, J. C. (1979). Anorexia nervosa in males. *The Lancet, 2,* 574–575.

Howe, J., Dickason, E. J., Jones, D. A., et al. (1984). *The Handbook of Nursing.* New York: John Wiley & Sons, Inc.

Kennedy-Caldwell, C. (1985). *Nutrition Support Nursing.* Silver Spring, MD: American Society for Parenteral and Enteral Nutrition.

Kim, M. J., McFarland, G. K., and McLane, A. M. (1984). *Pocket guide to nursing diagnoses.* St. Louis: C. V. Mosby Co.

Messner, R., and Lewis, S. (1984). Anorexia and bulimia: Disorders of mind and body. *Journal of the Society of Gastrointestinal Assistants, 7*(4), 8–14.
Rowland, C. J. (1984). *The monster within: Overcoming Bulimia.* Grand Rapids, MI: Baker Book House Co.
Sanger, E., and Cassino, L. (1984). Eating disorders: Avoiding the power struggle. *American Journal of Nursing, 84,* 31–35.
Zucker, P. (1984). *Eating disorders: Food for thought.* St. Louis: CMESat. Inc.

Chapter 10

The Patient with Alcoholism

Susan Lewis *William A. McDowell*
Robert J. Gregory *Roberta Messner*

I. STATEMENT OF PURPOSE

Alcoholism has been the topic of moral, religious, legal, and health-related concerns for centuries. It continues to be viewed by many as a sign of human weakness or personal failing rather than an illness. These challenging and frustrating patients are difficult to treat, and yet the potential for recovery is ever-present.

This chapter is designed for use by the nurse to:

- Increase understanding of the patient with alcohol problems.
- Facilitate nursing management by describing the care needed for the patient who is either acutely or chronically under the influence of alcohol.

II. OVERVIEW OF ALCOHOLISM

A. Description of the Illness

Alcoholism is a severe, progressive illness that will prove fatal if it is not arrested early enough in its course. An alcoholic can be defined as one who, because of alcohol consumption, has trouble

The authors wish to express special thanks to Alexander Nies, M.D., and Larry Smith, M.D., for their assistance in preparation of this manuscript.

Sections of this chapter are reprinted with permission of the Society of Gastrointestinal Assistants from the article:

Lewis, S., McDowell, W., Messner, R., Gregory, R., and Brown, J. (1985). Alcoholism: The problem behind the problem. *Journal of the Society of Gastrointestinal Assistants, 8*(2), 9–13 with family, job, society, health, and/or self. The criteria for diagnosis are based on the effects of alcohol on the person's life rather than how much or how often he drinks.

Some authorities classify alcoholism as the manifestation of a personality or behavior disorder associated with an unsatisfactory adjustment to life. Others believe that humans have a need to get "high" or to reach beyond the self for some greater experience.

Sometimes alcohol is used to cover serious psychological, emotional, or neurological symptoms. Alcoholism is said by some to be an inadequate means of coping. Although numerous theories have been proposed to explain alcoholism, the truth is that at this time no one knows why some people can drink socially and others, after one drink, cannot stop. Physiological and biochemical theories are being increasingly revived, and research is now intense. While there are still many more questions than answers, what is certain is that alcoholism is one of the several pharmacological addictions.

B. Incidence

Alcoholism is no respecter of persons, affecting all classes and races and posing a serious threat to the well-being of American society. The majority of alcoholics are respectable, intelligent people who maintain jobs. Only 5% of alcoholics are considered "skid-row bums" (Kinney and Leaton 1978).

Said to be the nation's third-largest health problem (Kaplan et al. 1980), alcoholism causes or contributes to such problems as gastrointestinal disease, organic brain syndrome, heart disease, burns, auto accidents, suicides, and homicides.

The National Institute of Alcoholism and Alcohol Abuse reports that 10%–15% of Americans are alcoholics or have problems related to alcohol (National Institute of Alcoholism and Alcohol Abuse 1983). The percentage of male alcoholics is approximately three times greater than that of female alcoholics, although the incidence of alcoholism seems to be increasing in females. It is estimated that approximately 3.3 million 14 to 17 year olds are problem drinkers (Stuart and Sundeen 1983). Alcoholism-related disorders constitute a large diagnostic category, and in some hospitals alcoholism ranks second only to heart disease (Stockford 1982). The Veterans Administration estimates that at least 50% of all Veterans Administration hospital beds are filled by veterans with alcohol problems (Kinney and Leaton 1978).

The alcoholic often engages in various forms of destructive behavior that affect the comfort and security of others. It has been estimated that each alcoholic, in some way, influences the lives of at least 8 to 13 other people.

C. Clinical Manifestations

1. General

One of the first effects of alcohol is to lessen inhibitions by depressing the inhibitory centers in the frontal lobes. This decreases self-criticism and judgment and produces a more comfortable feeling of self-confidence. Many alcoholics may develop antisocial characteristics, but few are outright sociopaths. Most feel inadequate and may be very dependent individuals. Drinking weakens inhibitions temporarily and allows freer expression of repressed desires. Excessive alcohol intake can precipitate a psychotic reaction.

Often the drinking pattern is cyclical in nature. Tension mounts, the individual drinks to resolve or lessen the tension, guilt occurs, fear of retaliation occurs, tension mounts, and the cycle begins again. Alcohol acts like an anesthetic. Feelings such as loneliness, guilt, insecurity, and fear are dissipated as the drinking continues. Resentment, however, does not seem to be affected because as inhibitions decrease, psychological controls also decrease. The individual may express negative thoughts and feelings that otherwise would not be expressed.

Early clues to alcoholism include: gulping drinks, development of tolerance, missing time from work (especially Monday), drinking alone, repeatedly requesting doctor's excuses for missing work for "stomach aches" or "colds," frequent drinking sprees, making excuses for drinking, irritability, shakiness in the morning, fatigue, blackouts, loss of appetite and weight change, insomnia, repeated accidents, poor and erratic work performance, drinking when upset, and using large amounts of coffee and cigarettes (Veterans Administration 1982). Later in the course of the illness morning drinking may occur.

Characteristics and symptoms of patients who are alcoholic may include the following:

a. Shaky, jittery, and weak
b. Insecure and resentful towards self, family, professionals, or authority figures
c. Hostile, demanding, rebellious, and critical
d. Inadequate, inferior, self-pitying, depressed, guilty, helpless, and hopeless
e. Lonely and isolated
f. Lacking in self respect
g. Often perfectionistic and intolerant of self and others
h. Fearful, distrustful, and somewhat paranoid
i. Often denies, minimizes and/or rationalizes drinking

j. Low tolerance for pain (emotional and physical) and frustration
k. Frequently overindulgent in oral satisfaction (e.g., smoking, eating, or medication)
l. Feels unloved and worthless
m. Often has a likeable and charming personality, though a somewhat superior facade
n. Usually does not wear well and frequently attempts to manipulate situations and people
o. Uncanny ability to bend regulations, split staff relations, and induce hostility in staff
p. Adept at maneuvering a significant person into the position of being "guilty" or the causative party for his or her drinking
q. Makes rules, then changes them to suit own purposes
r. Bends or ignores reality
s. Copes poorly with stress

2. Acute Intoxication

It is necessary to remember that there is approximately the same amount of alcohol in 10 oz of beer as in 6 oz of wine or 1 oz of 100-proof whiskey. While alcohol depresses the central nervous system to various degrees, the effects of alcohol and the duration of intoxication are dependent on the amount consumed, the rate of drinking, the amount and type of food in the stomach, body size, and that elusive intangible, tolerance.

Initially the behavioral effects are seen as "disinhibitory phenomena" (American Psychiatric Association 1980). Inhibitions may be reduced so that talk and emotional expression become easier. The individual may appear exceptionally bright, expansive, and hyperactive, with an increased sensation of well-being and mental acuity (American Psychiatric Association 1980).

As intoxication increases, the individual may develop a slowing of motor activity, with poor coordination and slowed

Table 10–1. COMMON PSYCHOSOCIAL MANIFESTATIONS OF ALCOHOLISM

Hostile, demanding, critical behavior, particularly toward authority figures
Depressed, hopeless affect
Diminished self-esteem
Often perfectionistic
Overindulgence in other areas (i.e., smoking, food, coffee, or medications)
Often has charistmatic personality but beneath this facade, feels worthless, inferior to others, guilty
Manipulative of people and situations
Low pain threshold
Poor coping skills

speech, and he may become withdrawn and dull. Impairment of judgment, intellectual activity, and memory occurs, as well as impairment in social and occupational functioning. Larger amounts produce altered perception and greater behavioral changes. Speech is slurred, unsteady gait and poor coordination may occur, nystagmus and flushing of the face may be noted, emotions may be erratic, and memory, judgment, and attention span are severely affected. Large doses can be lethal; however, loss of consciousness usually occurs before a lethal dose is consumed.

There is considerable individual variation in susceptibility to alcohol intoxication. Some individuals exhibit signs of intoxication with blood alcohol levels as low as 30mg %, while others do not appear intoxicated with blood levels as high as 150mg % (American Psychiatric Association 1980). Signs of intoxication are more evident when the blood alcohol level is rising than when it is falling. Most individuals will become intoxicated with blood alcohol levels of 100–200mg % (American Psychiatric Association 1980), with death being reported at levels varying from 400–700mg % (American Psychiatric Association 1980). The cause of death may be related to depression of respiration and/or aspiration of vomitus.

The gastrointestinal system is particularly susceptible to damage by alcohol ingestion. This is because the concentration of alcohol is far greater before it is absorbed than it is after being absorbed. Alcohol comes in direct contact with the stomach and intestinal lining, and can have a direct and even toxic effect.

The liver detoxifies alcohol at the rate of approximately 1–1½ oz per hour. Therefore, if an individual drinks a pint of whiskey, it takes his body 16 hours to detoxify the alcohol. Depending on the time of day that drinking begins, a person could still be under-the-influence on the next day.

3. Withdrawal Responses

Withdrawal symptoms seen during detoxification of the alcoholic patient range in severity from coarse tremor to grand mal seizures. Care of the patient in acute withdrawal and impending delirium tremens (DT's) is discussed below.

a. *Acute withdrawal* occurs within several hours after cessation or reduction in heavy, prolonged drinking of a duration of several days or longer. It begins with psychomotor agitation, commonly known as "the shakes." Other essential features include coarse tremor of the hands, tongue, and eyelids; nausea and vomiting; malaise or weakness; autonomic hyperactivity (tachycardia, diaphoresis, and increased blood pressure); anxiety; depressed mood; irritability; and orthostatic hypotension. Major motor seizures, known to the layman as "rum fits," are a serious complication and usually occur within 12 to 48 hours after cessation of drinking (Campbell and Frisse 1983). Withdrawal symptoms usually abate within 5–7 days unless alcohol withdrawal delirium (DT's) occurs (American Psychiatric Association 1980).

b. *Alcohol withdrawal delirium* (delirium tremens or DT's) is a condition often seen after someone has been drinking chronically for years. It usually occurs within 72–96 hours after the individual has stopped drinking or reduced the consumption of alcohol (Campbell and Frisse 1983). In some cases these symptoms may occur within a few hours after the last drink or as late as 10 days after cessation of drinking. Symptoms observed are coarse, irregular tremor, agitation, and autonomic hyperactivity, including fever. Delusions and vivid hallucinations, which are primarily visual but can occur in other sensory modalities, may be present. According to the *Diagnostic and Statistical Manual* of the American Psychiatric Association (1980), if seizures also occur as a result of alcohol withdrawal, they always precede the onset of delirium.

   DT's are considered a medical emergency, and there is a significant risk of death, with approximately a 20% death rate even among patients who receive treatment (Schultz and Dark 1986). Delirium often complicates other medical problems. A recovering surgical patient, for example, may be further imperiled by the manifestation of these symptoms.

c. *Alcohol hallucinosis* (American Psychiatric Association 1980) is an acute, although reversible, psychosis seen after prolonged excessive drinking of alcohol. It is characterized by the presence of vivid auditory hallucinations following reduction or cessation of drinking. It most often occurs within the first 48 hours after drinking has stopped (American Psychiatric Association 1980), but may occur up to 2 weeks after the last drink. The auditory hallucinations are usually voices that may speak to the individual directly, but most often discuss him or her in the third person. Frequently the content of these hallucinations is unpleasant, disturbing, and threatening. The individual may act to defend himself or herself by contacting the police or arming against intruders. Transient visual hallucinations may occur, as well as tremulousness, seizures, and in some cases, delirium. Ordinarily this disorder lasts only a few hours or days, and usually less than a week. In about 10% of cases it may last weeks or months, and in a few individuals a chronic form develops.

d. *Alcohol amnestic disorder* (American Psychiatric Association 1980) is a syndrome due to thiamine deficiency associated with prolonged, heavy use of alcohol. It often follows an acute episode of Wernicke's encephalopathy, which is a neurological disorder characterized by confusion, ataxia, eye-movement abnormalities, and other neurological signs. If symptoms of Wernicke's disease are treated early with large doses of thiamine, alcohol amnestic syndrome may be prevented.

   Alcohol amnestic disorder caused by thiamine deficiency is also known as Korsakoff's syndrome. Confabulation is the hallmark of Korsakoff's syndrome. It involves degeneration of both brain tissue and nerve endings. Symptoms include neurological disturbances such as peripheral neuropathy, cerebellar ataxia, myopathy, and major impairment of memory. Once alcohol amnestic disorder develops, it usually continues indefinitely. It can be quite severe, requiring lifelong custodial care.

e. *Dementia associated with alcoholism* (American Psychiatric Association 1980), or alcoholic deterioration, is seen after prolonged, excessive drinking in which vitamin deficiencies cause damage to brain tissue and nerve cells. Once the tissues are broken down, the damage is irreversible. Tenderness and pain over peripheral nerve endings may be noted. Severe burning pain on the soles of the feet may be present.

   The onset is gradual, and symptoms include a disintegration of personality. One of the initial symptoms is a tendency to act out impulsively. The individual develops feelings of guilt, resentment, irritability, and hostility, and may become careless in grooming. Affection is lost, perseverance and ambition disappear. This individual may appear congenial, euphoric, and in good humor to friends, but while at home, he may be a brutal tyrant. There is marked impairment in social and occupational functioning, and if the condition becomes severe, the individual may be oblivious to his environment.

f. The phenomenon referred to as *the "BUD" or "building-up to drink"* refers to increased vulnerability to resuming alcoholic drinking in response to some fairly predictable stress periods, especially during the first 2 years of sobriety.

However, BUDing may occur at any time during the life of the alcoholic. There are three times when the patient is especially vulnerable to "breaking over" during the first 2 years of sobriety. The first is during the 4th to 7th weeks of sobriety. The second occurs 4 to 7 weeks later. The third occurs after 11 to 13 months of sobriety. Close observation reveals that the alcoholic shows signs of confusion and frustration days or even weeks before "breaking over" for the next drink. Often the family can notice these symptoms before the patient is aware of them. Some believe that the symptoms of this emotional discomfort may be caused by physical agitation. The pattern is usually cyclic, and symptoms begin and progress slowly. Moodiness, irritability, boredom, and restlessness are noted, as well as complaints of physical discomfort. As tension builds over days or weeks, the patient is likely to resume drinking.

III. NURSING MANAGEMENT

A. Assessment

Assessment of drinking behavior should be a part of the nursing history on *every* patient. Alcoholics tend to minimize drinking, insisting, "I can take it or leave it," or to deny drinking altogether. One standard patient response is, "I had just a couple of drinks," covering the fact that he lost count after a couple. If alcoholism is suspected, it is wise to include the family in the history-taking process. The family may talk more freely if allowed the opportunity to speak privately in a separate room.

Drinking history should include:

1. Age at first drink.
2. Length of time drinking has been a problem.
3. Patterns of drinking, that is, does the patient drink daily or does he drink in binges?
4. Effects of drinking behavior on the patient's life, whether family problems, legal problems, employment problems, health problems such as GI disturbances or liver disease, or social problems.
5. Assessment for alcohol blackouts, those periods of time when drinking for which the patient has no memory.
6. History of delirium tremens or alcohol hallucinosis.
7. Record of depressive episodes or suicide attempts.
8. Time of last drink—this is crucial in observation for monitoring withdrawal and DT's.

9. Patient's own definition of alcoholism.
10. Willingness to admit he has a problem.
11. Willingness to accept help and treatment.
12. Presence or absence of patient strengths, available support systems, and resources.
13. Use of other means of oral gratification such as cigarettes and coffee. (Nicotine and caffeine are also pharmacologically addicting chemicals.)

B. Planning

Planning of nursing care for the alcoholic patient should be based on a comprehensive nursing assessment and subsequent nursing diagnosis.

Alcoholics are heavy consumers of the services provided by the health care system. Accordingly, they will be found in virtually all programs, including outpatient clinics, inpatient hospital services, and specialized units such as psychiatric hospitals and alcoholic treatment programs (ATPs). Treatment necessarily includes detoxification, intensive education and rehabilitation programs, and long-term convalescence with continuing care.

For those addicted to alcohol, the nurse can recommend detoxification, immediately followed by an intensive treatment program and continued long-term followup. Frequently the recommendation is adopted only through pressure from family members, employers, or the legal system. For those who are detoxified, an intensive treatment program should immediately follow the detoxification period. During this time, a treatment team of medical, psychological, and social work professionals will seek to enable the patient to regain physical health, understand the emotional and affective aspects and consequences of alcoholism, and straighten out the often tangled web of family relationships. Discharge to the family and community generally requires continued support and intervention when relapses occur. Modification of the plan should be carried out based on reassessments of the progress of the patient and evaluation of the care given.

It is useful to set short- and long-term goals with the alcoholic patient.

1. Short-term goals include:
    a. Provide a safe detoxification period and control of the symptoms of delirium tremens and other withdrawal responses.
    b. Help the patient realize that the immediate goal is remaining abstinent, one day at a time.
    c. Help the patient realize that he has a problem with alcohol.

d. Provide acceptable methods of relieving tension and anxiety other than escape with alcohol.
e. Help the patient tolerate frustration and feelings of loneliness and helplessness.
f. Begin rehabilitation as soon as the patient is admitted to the hospital for alcoholism.

2. Long-term goals include helping the patient:
   a. Realize that the primary goal is lasting, total abstinence.
   b. Realize that many of his active problems are secondary to drinking and that alcoholism is a lifelong illness. Assure the patient that his or her life can and must be managed without alcohol.
   c. Discover new, more positive ways to meet personal needs.
   d. Regain self-respect and self-confidence.
   e. Discover more positive ways of coping with stress and frustration.
   f. Understand anxiety and depression and when and where to seek help.
   g. Seek new ways of feeling pleasure.

C. Intervention

1. Prevention

The purpose of prevention is to decrease the incidence of individuals who develop alcohol problems. Efforts to prevent alcoholism have had little or no success thus far. It is apparent that "preaching the evils of alcohol and the dangers of alcoholism is ineffective" (Kinney and Leaton 1978).

Education is a vital component in informing individuals about the illness of alcoholism. Responsible drinking behavior has been the focus of educational efforts and mass media advertising. Whether or not these endeavors are successful will have to be evaluated in the future.

Great stigma is still attached to alcoholics and alcoholism. Education attempts to change these attitudes. Factual information about the drug alcohol, the disease of alcoholism, and where to find help should be included. It should be emphasized that alcoholism is a disease with recognizable signs and symptoms, and that it can be successfully treated. In addition, alcohol education should stress self-awareness, management of guilt feelings and low self-esteem, and taking responsibility for one's actions.

Children of alcoholics are of great concern. Recent research and observation has shown that children of alcoholics not only are more vulnerable to the illness of alcoholism as adults, but also suffer lasting effects from growing up in a dysfunctional, alcoholic family. The need for education, treatment, and continued research with this population is monumental. The nurse can have a powerful role in identifying these people, providing education, and encouraging treatment.

2. Treatment

   Effective nursing management involves assessment, short- and long-term planning, intervention both during acute phases and over long-term convalescence, and evaluation. In managing the treatment of alcoholism, the authors recommend the 5 a's: Attitude, Abstinence, Alcohol Treatment Programs, Alcoholics Anonymous, and Antabuse.

   a. *Attitude* is crucial to treatment. Denial is a strong defense mechanism used by alcoholics. Unless the alcoholic recognizes and admits a problem, treatment is ineffective. The attitude of the staff is also important. Staff members with negative attitudes toward alcoholics will definitely hinder treatment.
   b. *Abstinence* from alcohol is crucial. The patient cannot drink. The old saying that "once an alcoholic, always an alcoholic" seems appropriate. Some clinicians still hold the theory that alcoholics can learn to drink safely in social situations; however the authors of this chapter and most researchers have not found this to be true.
   c. *Alcoholic Treatment Programs* (ATPs) are available through federal, state, local, and private facilities. The majority of these programs are residential and last 4 to 6 weeks. These programs provide education and group and individual therapy. They also afford the patient an extended number of days free from alcohol and a chance to look at himself and his problems and find new ways to cope. This extended period provides an opportunity for the alcoholic to "dry out" and clear some of his or her mental confusion. After discharge from an ATP, the patient still needs to continue involvement in an outpatient treatment program for a prolonged period.
   d. *Alcoholics Anonymous* (AA) is an organization available to all alcoholics and their families. It claims one of the best success rates of all types of alcohol treatment. It is nonresidential and is available in every area of the country. A frequent recommendation is that the alcoholic attend 90 meetings in 90 days. AA helps structure time that used to be spent drinking and provides an emotional support system.

e. *Antabuse* (disulfiram) is a medication taken daily to serve as a deterrent to drinking. It causes few, if any, side effects unless combined with alcohol. Antabuse inhibits an enzyme that normally removes toxic products of alcohol metabolism. Therefore, if the patient drinks while taking antabuse, he will become violently ill with nausea and vomiting, throbbing in the head and neck, flushing of the face, hyperventilation, and hypotension. It is estimated that 1 in 1000 people who drink while on Antabuse will die from the reaction. Antabuse remains in the system for up to 14 days. Therefore, if antabuse patients plan to drink, they have to wait 10–14 days after the last dose before it is safe to do so. Hopefully, during that waiting period, they will change their minds. Counseling may also be helpful.

Dosages of 250 mg per day will provide a maintenance level, although 500 mg may be used initially. A few select patients may be maintained on 500 mg per day. Side effects are few, minor, and rare. However, Antabuse is contraindicated if there is impaired judgment, cardiovascular disease, and liver or kidney failure. The patient should be cautioned against giving blood while on Antabuse. A medical review should be required before use, and the patient must be fully informed about the consequences of the effects. Antabuse is a tool, not a magical treatment nor a substitute for a comprehensive program of recovery.

3. Medications

During detoxification, the benzodiazepines are useful since they are cross-tolerant with alcohol and allow a safer, more predictable detoxification. However, they are not recommended in treatment following detoxification because they are similar in effect to alcohol and may themselves lead to addiction. Major tranquilizers are sometimes useful in treating anxiety, but not for the treatment of alcoholism. Antidepressants may be useful in reducing depression in a small number of select patients. Thiamine and magnesium sulfate should be given to replace these nutrients and to help prevent seizure activity and brain damage.

Antabuse (disulfiram) is used to deter alcohol consumption, as noted previously.

4. Nursing Actions

a. Acute withdrawal and impending delirium tremens

- Because many people have negative feelings toward alcoholism and alcoholics, and these feelings can interfere with treatment, it is essential that the nurse be attuned to her personal feelings toward alcoholism and alcoholics.

Strong (particularly negative) "countertransference" feelings are toxic to both patient and nurse.

- Recovery begins only when the patient recognizes and admits that he has a problem; the patient should be encouraged to recognize and admit that his alcohol use generates problems and is out of control.
- During withdrawal, the patient may become combative and destructive to get away from tormentors, snakes, and bugs that may be felt or sensed as crawling on his skin. Patients may be suicidal. Provide a safe, protective, supervised environment for the patient who is confused, disoriented, and hallucinating. The patient detoxifying from alcohol can be extremely disruptive on a medical-surgical unit.
- Keep the environment lighted to decrease sensory illusions that may augment anxiety and cause hallucinations. Decrease shadows, which the patient may interpret as small animals on clothing, bedding, or walls.
- Keep surroundings as quiet as possible, since loud noises may increase anxiety and agitation.
- Keep windows closed and locked, for if the patient believes he is being followed, pursued, or chased, jumping from a window may be regarded as an appropriate escape route.
- Use physical restraints only when necessary, for they may aggravate restlessness and make the patient feel imprisoned. Physical restraints are sometimes necessary for the patient's safety.
- Keep the bed in a low position with rails up to prevent jumping or falling from the bed.
- Observe the patient closely for symptoms of impending DT's or seizures. Patients can go into DT's up to 10 days after the last drink. DT's is a potentially fatal condition and is considered a medical emergency.
- Force fluids, especially fruit juices. Give vitamins and a high-caloric, high-protein diet. Encourage snacking. Use decaffeinated coffee. The patient is often dehydrated and in poor nutritional status. Physical and nutritional rehabilitation are necessary, since alcoholism destroys physical health.
- Help with feeding if tremors are so severe that they interfere with the use of hands.
- Promote sleep and rest, with warm showers at night, hot drinks, and drugs prescribed to sedate during withdrawal. Allow the patient to sleep as long as possible. Alcohol

and alcohol withdrawal interfere with normal sleep patterns. Rest and sleep can make detoxification less unpleasant. Benzodiazepines and other drugs can help decrease the risk of DT's.

- Observe vital signs. Record input and output during detoxification to provide clues to potential problem situations.
- Treat the patient fairly, but be alert to his efforts to get special attention, bypass hospital rules, or seek special favors. The alcoholic patient may be unreliable and persuasive.
- Explain reasons for all tests and procedures to gain more cooperation and reduce the patient's fear of not knowing what is happening.
- Assist the patient when out of bed during withdrawal period or when heavily sedated. The patient may be shaky and unsteady during withdrawal. Falls are likely during this period, as well as when heavily sedated.
- Allow the patient to talk about problems, to express feelings of resentment, hopelessness, guilt, and remorse, and to express rationalizations and alibis. Listen with respect, for alcoholism causes multiple problems for the patient.

b. Continuing treatment and convalescence

- Understand that alcoholism is a progressive illness that can be arrested. Enable the patient to understand the nature of this illness and to admit to being an alcoholic.
- Accept the patient as a worthwhile human being. Although the alcoholic has increased feelings of shame, guilt, and worthlessness, do not reinforce these feelings. The individual needs to learn self-worth and dignity.
- Plan regular daily routines to provide an adequate balance of rest, work, socialization, and interaction with others. Patients are usually in poor physical and nutritional health, and need to learn to re-establish healthful patterns of living.
- Look for symptoms of depression, which is an aftermath of withdrawal. Chronic, underlying depression is frequently found in many alcoholics.
- Observe for symptoms of underlying mental illness, since some cases of alcoholism are a result of mental illness in which the patient is self-treating symptoms with alcohol.
- Encourage the patient to make personal decisions to cope with life's responsibilities without using alcohol. Teach problem-solving skills. Permanent rehabilitation is

facilitated by the patient's decision to quit using alcohol as an emotional crutch.

- Confront the patient who manipulates. The alcoholic is often a con artist, skilled at flattering staff to obtain favors and talented at obtaining special privileges or getting staff to overlook infractions of rules.
- Insist that the patient complete tasks or work assignments. Completing small responsibilities facilitates progression to greater ones. One treatment goal is to aid the alcoholic in meeting responsibilities without alcohol.
- Be firm, yet helpful and understanding. Rejection or perceived rejection from staff inhibits treatment.
- Allow the patient to ventilate anger and hostility. The alcoholic feels guilt, anger, and resentment. Expression of these feelings helps the patient deal with them.
- Encourage physical participation in recreational activity. Activity promotes physical health and helps the patient learn to interact with others. It also helps disseminate feelings of frustration and anger.
- Formulate a treatment plan and be consistent. Do not allow the patient to play one staff member against another. The alcoholic does not like authority, rules, and regulations. He often takes reality and twists it to cause embarrassment or animosity in those he is trying to use.
- Give emotional support without being overly sympathetic to the patient. Use a firm, kind, calm, matter-of-fact manner with the patient to prevent manipulation and to discourage the alcoholic from attempting to gain favors or make excuses for his condition.
- Do not accept the patient's explanations and reassurances when he minimizes his drinking problem or brags about exploits. The alcoholic can cleverly camouflage problems and behavior with rationalization and minimization. Use a neutral attitude. At times, the alcoholic superficially seems so rational, but the illness has an irrational or nonrational basis. Be careful to listen to not only what you are hearing, but also what you are not hearing.
- Encourage the alcoholic to tone down superior attitudes, which are often defense mechanisms used to hide real feelings of guilt, shame, and inadequacy. Sometimes a superior attitude is used as an excuse to deny being an alcoholic and avoid working in treatment.
- Help the patient focus on strengths and talents. Stressing the patient's worth and positive traits helps build a positive self-image.

- Spend time with the patient when he is convalescing to allay loneliness. The alcoholic has deep, unsatisfied needs for love, power, and prestige for which there is little chance of fulfilling.
- Provide diversions. Too much unstructured time is a hinderance to recovery. Without alcohol, the patient often does not know what to do with time.
- Welcome the patient each time he presents for treatment, whether drunk or sober, and regardless of the number of times. Relapses are common and are often a necessary part of the patient's education. Each relapse is a reminder that the only path is continued abstinence.
- Accept the admission of alcoholism in a kind, nonjudgmental way. Successful treatment of the alcoholic cannot be accomplished by rejecting attitudes from therapeutic personnel.
- Refer the patient to AA and encourage the use of ATPs, Antabuse, and community resources. Encourage family members to attend Al Anon. Telephone numbers of AA are listed in every directory. AA has members available to talk with alcoholics or their families and to provide transportation to meetings. Alcoholism should never be considered cured, but can be arrested. Continued treatment and followup are necessary. The family also requires education and treatment.
- Emphasize to the patient that he is worth saving. Many alcoholics have self-destructive tendencies and seek through drink an oblivion to escape from reality and situations with which they cannot cope.
- Encourage the patient to help others with the same problems. Helping others with this problem provides strength, reinforcement, and satisfaction to the recovering alcoholic.
- As recovery occurs, make the patient increasingly responsible for himself. The primary treatment goal is to help the patient meet life's responsibilities and learn effective ways of coping without alcohol. This begins with small responsibilities—such as keeping appointments, maintaining personal hygiene, and preparing meals—and progresses to greater responsibilities, such as maintaining a job or coping with disappointment or a family crisis.

D. Evaluation/Expected Outcomes

Effective nursing management can be evaluated in terms of the following criteria.

1. The nurse will:
   a. Provide an emotionally warm and stable environment.
   b. Meet the physical (physiological) needs of the patient until he can do this.
   c. Gradually increase the levels of responsibility to be handled by the patient.
   d. Recognize and deal with negative thoughts and feelings about the alcoholic patient.
2. The patient will:
   a. Learn, realize, and understand the facts of alcoholism and accept these facts as being self-applicable. This includes the admission of being an alcoholic
   b. Cease all use of alcohol and other sedative drugs.
   c. Learn and practice constructive use of time.
   d. Take increasing responsibility for the activities of daily living.
   e. Interact with staff and other patients, family, and friends. Join AA.
   f. Identify and evaluate feelings, behaviors, and situations that precipitate drinking behavior, including "BUD," and seek to bring about appropriate personal changes.
   g. Identify and verbalize personal strengths. Build a positive self-image.

E. Evaluation for Referral

Alcoholic patients who recognize and admit their problem and are willing to seek treatment should be referred to Alcoholics Anonymous (AA) or an alcohol treatment program (ATP) following detoxification. ATPs are residential programs lasting approximately 21–28 days. After completing an ATP the patient should be referred to AA or other community support groups for extended followup. Families should be referred to Al Anon.

IV. POTENTIAL NURSING DIAGNOSES

1. Coping, ineffective, related to
   - impaired thought processes
   - anger
   - low frustration tolerance
   - dependency needs
   - inadequate skills for management of stressors

2. Injury, potential for, related to
   - altered thought processes
   - low self-esteem
   - suidical ideation
   - anger
   - effects of chemical use
3. Self-care deficit, related to
   - low self-esteem
   - disinterest
   - impaired thought processes
4. Self-concept, alterations in, related to
   - poor self-esteem
   - depression
   - physiological effects of alcohol
   - guilt
5. Violence, potential for, related to
   - impaired judgment
   - effects of chemical use
   - lack of impulse control
   - impaired physical functioning
   - impaired perception and mental acuity

V. SUMMARY

It is difficult for the average person to comprehend the struggle an alcoholic has in achieving sobriety. It is more than a matter of just deciding not to drink. The old adage "once an alcoholic, always an alcoholic" appears to hold true. An alcoholic cannot and should not drink socially. An alcoholic may maintain 20 years of sobriety only to find that if he tries to drink again, the same or even worse results follow.

In caring for the alcoholic patient, what seems kindest may not help him and may hinder treatment or actually facilitate drinking behavior. *Permitting avoidance of the real problem, the drinking, because of anger or because it is easier to ignore the problem altogether does not allow the alcoholic to realize there is a problem.* Confrontation may be upsetting, but until the patient realizes and admits that he is an alcoholic, the first step on the road to recovery cannot be taken.

Treatment is both frustrating and rewarding. To be effective, the nurse must be aware of personal feelings about alcoholism and alcoholics. If the nurse has negative feelings toward the alcoholic patient, this can interfere with the ability to give effective care. Not everyone can work with alcoholics. Many people still regard alcoholism as a human failing, not as an illness. It is disheartening to work diligently with a patient, only to witness a relapse. And yet, relapses are common with alcoholics and are often a necessary part of the patient's education. Each relapse, or "fall off the wagon," reinforces the fact that he cannot drink and further serves as a reminder that continued abstinence is mandatory. In fact, the alcoholic's very survival depends on it.

References

American Psychiatric Association (1980). *Diagnostic and statistical manual of mental disorders* (3rd ed.). Washington, DC: American Psychiatric Association.

Campbell, J. W., and Frisse, M. (Ed.). (1983). *Manual of medical therapeutics* (3rd ed.). Boston: Little, Brown and Company; St. Louis: Department of Medicine, Washington University School of Medicine.

Clunn, P. A., and Payne, B. P. (1982). *Psychiatric mental health nursing* (3rd ed.). Garden City, NY: Medical Examination Publishing Co., Inc.

Crawford, A. L., and Kilander, V. C. (1980). *Psychiatric nursing: A basic manual.* Philadelphia: F. A. Davis Company.

Kaplan, H. I., Freedman, A. M., and Sadock, B. J. (1980). *Comprehensive textbook of psychiatry* (3rd ed., Vol. 2). Baltimore: Williams & Wilkins Co.

Kinney, J., and Leaton, G. (1978). *Loosening the grip.* St. Louis: C. V. Mosby Company.

Lewis, S., McDowell, W., Messner, R., et al. (1985). Alcoholism: The problem behind the problem. *Journal of the Society of Gastrointestinal Assistants, 8*(2), 9–13.

National Institute of Alcoholism and Alcohol Abuse (1983). Personal communication.

Schultz, J. M., and Dark, S. L. (1986). *Manual of psychiatric nursing care plans* (2nd ed.). Boston: Little, Brown and Company.

Stockford, D. (1982). *1980 Supplement to alcoholism and problem drinking, 1970–1975. A statistical analysis of VA hospital patients.* Washington, DC: Statistical Policy and Research Service Office of Reports and Statistics, Veterans Administration.

Stuart, G. W., and Sundeen, S. J. (1983). *Principles and practice of psychiatric nursing.* St. Louis: C. V. Mosby Company.

Veterans Administration (1982). *Program guide—Nursing service* (G-10, M-2, Part V). Washington, DC: U.S. Government Printing Office.

Chapter 11

The Patient with Drug Dependence

Susan Lewis *Theodore B. Feldmann*

I. STATEMENT OF PURPOSE

Drug addiction is a disease that is progressive, predictable, and potentially fatal (Smith and Wesson, 1985). Nursing care of addicted patients is complex and requires a consistent team approach. The success rate for recovery is limited and the potential for relapse is great. The purpose of this chapter is:

- To introduce the nurse to the drug-dependent patient.
- To offer guidelines for nursing care.

II. OVERVIEW OF DRUG DEPENDENCE AND ABUSE

A. Description of the Illness

Addictive disease is multidimensional, encompassing physical, psychosocial, pharmacological, behavioral, and spiritual factors. The disease process is progressive and pathological with characteristic signs and symptoms. The prognosis is predictable and potentially fatal. Symptoms vary in complexity depending on the progression of the disease.

The Diagnostic and Statistical Manual (DSM-III-R) of the American Psychiatric Association divides substance use disorders into two categories: substance abuse and substance dependence. Substance abuse includes a pattern of pathological use, impairment of occupational or social functioning, and a brief duration of at least one month. Substance abuse can take many forms, including misuse of prescription medication. Some authorities believe that drug abuse occurs anytime a drug is taken in a manner other than that prescribed.

According to the DSM-III-R, substance dependence occurs

when tolerance to the drug develops, requiring ever-increasing doses to produce the desired effect; when withdrawal symptoms occur when the drug is not taken; and after a duration of at least one month. A functional definition is offered by Smith and Wesson (1985), who define dependence as a compulsion to use a drug, loss of control over the amount used, and continued use despite adverse consequences.

B. Incidence

The misuse and abuse of psychoactive drugs has reached epidemic proportions in this country. Because a significant number of Americans are involved with at least occasional use of drugs, this constitutes a major health problem.

The use of drugs by adolescents and even children is the focus of extensive media coverage. Drug use occurs at all levels of society, with an ever-increasing popularity among middle and upper classes. Indeed, many of our modern-day heroes, such as athletes and entertainers, are known to be drug users.

The majority of drug users never come to the attention of health care providers. Those who do often have histories of using drugs to cope with unresolved conflicts, feelings of depression, serious personality disturbances, or other psychiatric problems. These individuals often have severe medical problems and/or are in serious legal trouble. Patients with severe personality disorders are at increased risk for developing drug dependence.

The illicit use of drugs is greatest in the 18- to 25-year-old age group and is the leading cause of death in this group (Crawford and Kilander 1980). Although the number of heroin addicts is said to have decreased in recent years, the annual death rate of opiate-dependent people was reported by the American Psychiatric Association as 10 per 1000 in 1980.

Cocaine is currently one of the most popular and dangerous drugs being abused in the United States. According to *Time Magazine,* conservative estimates indicate that 10 million Americans use cocaine regularly, and an additional 5 million have used it experimentally (Delmarest 1981).

Psychoactive prescription drugs and tranquilizers are the most frequently abused of all prescription medications. Women are the greatest users of drugs in this category. In 1979 the Surgeon General estimated that at least 1,000,000 Americans abuse sedative-hypnotics, with approximately 30,000 being addicted to them (Bennett et al. 1983). The most common form of nonmedical use of sedative-hypnotics or tranquilizers is the occasional pill borrowed from a friend or relative for nervousness or sleep.

Individuals over age 55 are the largest consumers of legal drugs. The task force on prescription drugs found that the average person over age 65 acquired about three times as many prescription drugs in all categories and spent about three times as much money for drugs as younger people (Bennett et al. 1983).

In children and adolescents, use of any psychoactive drug alone or in combination poses serious health hazards.

Caffeine, nicotine, and alcohol remain the most commonly used mood-altering drugs. Although there are no statistics on the number of adult Americans who have *never* used a mood-altering drug, the number would appear to be slight.

C. Clinical Manifestations*

The life of the drug-dependent individual is consumed with the craving to achieve an alteration in mood or level of consciousness by using one or more chemical agents. Because obtaining the drug may be expensive, criminal behavior often compounds the addict's list of problems. In short, the addict does not control the drug, it controls him.

These individuals seem to have a low tolerance for any type of discomfort, either physical or emotional. The habitual use of mood-altering drugs deadens the senses and allows temporary escape. The drug produces a transient feeling of well-being with all needs being met.

Drug-dependent persons are often emotionally immature, passive, dependent, and at times self-destructive. They use drugs to satisfy oral needs and often avoid or are incapable of sexual experiences. Drugs may also be used to fill certain deficits in the personality.

Nurses need to be aware that patients with chronic pain and/or extreme anxiety may be vulnerable to dependence on prescription drugs. Clues to dependence can include requesting the medication more frequently than ordered, repeated excuses that the medication has been stolen or damaged, and signs of intoxication. It is important and very often difficult to distinguish between those patients suffering from intense pain and those patients who are dependent on their medication. Patients with chronic pain need medication to help alleviate the pain. For these patients, drugs that are not habit-forming or that potentiate the action of narcotics should be considered, as well as techniques such as biofeedback, autogenic relaxation, and visual imagery.

Drug-dependent patients are often untruthful, misleading, and

---

*See Appendix D, "Table of Psychoactive Drugs," for information on specific drugs.

insincere with their own hidden agendas. Behavior can vary from excessive activity to apathy. These patients often want things their own way, and become demanding and threatening when this is denied. They tend to blame others for all of their problems and take little responsibility for their own behavior. They are highly manipulative and very adept at using others for their own advantage. Drug addicts often behave in a clever and beguiling manner in an attempt to charm and manipulate the staff. Unsuspecting staff often feel sorry for these individuals and at times grant them special favors.

Acutely intoxicated behavior is easily identified. The following symptoms may be noted:

1. Impaired sensorium
2. Impaired judgment
3. Ataxia
4. Slurred speech
5. Bizarre behavior
6. Poor grooming and hygiene
7. Odor of alcohol on breath
8. Odor of marihuana on clothing and hair

Chronic substance users may be more difficult to recognize on the basis of observable signs, particularly between episodes of acute intoxication. Fresh needle marks on arms, legs, or neck would be an observable clue. Taking a careful history is essential in identifying chronic users.

In the workplace assessment of absenteeism, deterioration of job skills, reduced productivity, and theft may give clues to drug addiction.

III. NURSING MANAGEMENT

A. Assessment

Many drug-dependent patients who present for treatment are in some crisis or are forced into treatment by the courts. Drug-dependent patients are often polysubstance abusers. The more drugs used in combination with each other, the more chaotic the patient's behavior. Other complications can be related to the substance used to cut, or dilute, drugs that are sold on the streets.

Because of these and other factors, a thorough assessment is crucial. It is not uncommon for these patients to give false information and omit details on initial evaluation. Careful assessment must be ongoing throughout treatment in order to obtain a complete history. It is extremely beneficial to interview family and significant others as well.

Assessment should include:

1. Psychosocial history
2. Current life stressors
3. Identification of cultural influences
4. Reasons for seeking treatment. (Often the patient has serious health problems or legal charges, or his supplier is no longer available.)
5. Drugs currently being used—types, amounts, and frequency of usage. (The drug patient may exaggerate or underestimate amounts used.)
6. Drugs used in the past
7. Pattern of use
8. How does the patient support the habit?
9. How does the patient see the world and his place in it?
10. How does the patient handle responsibility?
11. Job-holding skills
12. Ability to form and sustain relationships
13. Defense mechanisms and coping skills
14. Motivation for treatment—how serious is he?
15. Health status—nutrition, infection, and so on.
16. Current and past legal problems
17. Sexual history
18. Family history of substance abuse

A complete psychiatric evaluation to rule out underlying psychiatric problems or personality disorders should be obtained after the patient has been detoxified and has maintained sobriety for a period of time. Many of the symptoms of psychiatric and social disturbances may be related to the effects of the drug itself or the lifestyle of the drug culture.

B. Planning

Following a thorough nursing assessment, planning for care will be based on the individual needs of the patient. *Continuity of care is crucial in treating drug-dependent patients.*

Although the patient should be included in the formulation of the treatment plan, this should be done with careful consideration. Drug-dependent patients often have hidden agendas and will attempt to dictate their own treatment. For example, a drug addict approached a nurse claiming that he wanted to "get off" drugs. After speaking with him briefly, it became clear that he was asking to be detoxified from dilaudid, but wanted to continue use of codeine, valium, and phenobarbital. A similar situation is often seen with the patients who combine cocaine, alcohol, and marihuana. They may see cocaine as a problem and wish to be detoxified, but may not even mention alcohol and marihuana use because these are not viewed as part of the problem.

Treatment for drug-dependent patients should be realistic. Often they are not able to see that what is best for them is different from what they desire. These patients are frequently unwilling to suffer any discomfort during the treatment process.

C. Intervention

1. Prevention

Education is an essential element in prevention of drug abuse and dependence. It should begin at home with the very young child. Parents with the ability to demonstrate healthy coping behavior without reliance on drugs have a powerful influence.

Drug education should be offered in the primary grades and continue throughout school. Teaching problem-solving and effective, alternative coping skills can help prevent drug use. Young people can be taught skills necessary to resist the pressure to use mood-altering chemicals. Assertiveness training and self-management as alternatives to drug use for recreation, reduction of anxiety, and excitement can be included in this type of program.

The mass media can exert a powerful effect, especially on youth. The visibility of popular figures who demonstrate healthy behavior in relation to substance use can counteract negative role-modeling.

The employment setting is another arena in which attempts to prevent substance abuse and dependence can take place. Employers can provide both education and intervention programs for employees. The desire to maintain one's job can be an excellent motivator in seeking treatment. Also, the prospect of getting a job or learning a skill to make employment possible can be an incentive for relapse prevention for those who are unemployed.

2. Treatment*

Permanent rehabilitation of the drug addict is highly influenced by his personal commitment to be free of addiction. The addict needs to adopt a drug-free philosophy of life fully. Recovery is much more than withdrawal; it involves embracing a new lifestyle.

Treatment and recovery are based on a continuum of phases:

---

*See Appendix D, "Table of Psychoactive Drugs," for information on specific drugs.

a. Withdrawal/detoxification
b. Long-term residential treatment
c. On-going after-care outpatient followup through recovery groups
d. Education and treatment of codependents

The care approach to treatment is based on the peer group/therapeutic community concept. Often ex-addicts provide strong role-model identification. The treatment environment should offer organization, structure, and control. Rules and regulations should be clearly communicated. Consequences of infractions should be enforced.

A multidisciplinary team providing consistency of care is essential.

Programs for adult children of alcoholics, Narcotics Anonymous, and Al Anon are also valuable.

3. Medications

Unfortunately, the personality structure of some opiate addicts is so defective that they are never able to function without the emotional support provided by the drug. An alternative for these individuals is methadone maintenance. Methadone itself is an addicting drug with a duration of action of 24–36 hours. It can be taken once a day and will prevent withdrawal symptoms from opiates. It is said to block "the rush" or intense high that injecting heroin gives. Patients on methadone are able to function in society and work. They should continue in group therapy on a regular basis. Strict government regulations control the use of methadone for detoxification and maintenance.

Clonidine is a drug sometimes used as an adjunct to detoxification from opiates. It has been found to prevent the sympathetic hyperactivity experienced during opiate withdrawal. Sluggishness and hypotension have been reported as side effects when clonidine is used in this manner.

Narcan (naloxone) is an opiate antagonist that can be used in emergency situations to counteract respiratory depression. Nalline (nalorphine) also rapidly overcomes respiratory depression induced by opiates. These drugs are sometimes used in diagnosis of narcotic dependence. Administration of Narcan or Nalline will produce mild withdrawal symptoms in an addicted patient.

4. Nursing Actions
   a. Be aware of personal feelings about working with drug-dependent patients
   b. A multidisciplinary team approach is essential

c. Be consistent—these patients will attempt to manipulate staff to their own ends.
d. Communicate regulations clearly and ahead of time.
e. Enforce rules consistently.
f. Observe the patient for signs of withdrawal, including convulsions.
g. Monitor vital signs.
h. Use palliative measures to ease the physical discomfort of muscle spasms and twitching (sometimes termed "kicking the habit"). Intense leg cramps accompany withdrawal and may be experienced for months thereafter.
i. One-to-one supportive encounters should be brief and focus on physical symptoms.
j. Be friendly and supportive while maintaining a therapeutic distance.
k. Be aware of the patient's ability to be charming and beguiling in order to manipulate.
l. Be truthful and concise.
m. Assist the patient in finding more productive ways to deal with anxiety and discomfort.
n. Search incoming items such as food and clothing for drugs; some patients have been known to sprinkle powdered drugs on potato chips or conceal alcohol in cola cans.
o. Observe the patient for depression and suicidal ideation.
p. Personally observe the patient taking any medication prescribed for him.
q. Check for needle tracks and treat infections or other physical complications.
r. Random, observed urine screens should be taken.
s. Use blood and body fluid precautions on all patients to prevent the spread of infectious diseases such as hepatitis and AIDS. According to the Surgeon General, 17% of AIDS patients are intravenous drug abusers.
t. Disciplinary discharge may be used for infractions of the rules.
u. Overnight and weekend passes should be used sparingly or not al all.

D. Evaluation/Expected Outcomes

Effective nursing management can be evaluated in terms of observable behaviors.

1. The nurse will:
   a. Provide guidance and support for the patient as he progresses through withdrawal and treatment

b. Promote independence and responsibility in the patient.

2. The patient will:
   a. Be honest with himself and others.
   b. Assume responsibility for his own behavior.
   c. Maintain a drug-free existence.
   d. Adopt a more productive lifestyle.
   e. Change self-destructive or maladaptive behavior.
   f. Increase independence.
   g. Request assistance from others when needed.
   h. Establish a support system apart from drug or alcohol users.
   i. Demonstrate social skills that increase self-awareness and self-esteem.
   j. Continue in therapy on an on-going basis.

E. Evaluation for Referral

Drug-dependent patients should be confronted about their drug behavior. This may be most appropriately done by professionals who work in drug treatment. The detoxification phase may occur on a medical-surgical unit, on a psychiatric unit, or as part of a drug treatment program. The opportunity for referral to a drug treatment program (DTP) should be offered. These are residential programs that are from 1 month to 2 years in duration and involve intensive individual and group therapy. After discharge from a DTP, patients should be referred to followup in community-based organizations such as Narcotics Anonymous.

IV. POTENTIAL NURSING DIAGNOSES

1. Anxiety, related to
   - lifestyle
   - drug dependence
   - anger
   - physical effects of the drugs
   - mood changes due to drug use
   - withdrawal symptoms
   - impaired judgment and thought processes
2. Coping, ineffective individual, related to
   - dependence on drugs
   - poor interpersonal skills
   - dependency needs
   - low frustration tolerance

3. Self-care deficit, related to significant change in habits, activities of daily living, self-care activities, and level of independence.
4. Self-concept, alterations in, related to
   - dependence on drugs
   - poor self-esteem
   - guilt

V. SUMMARY

Drug dependence is difficult to treat, and the rates of recidivism are high. Recovery is not accomplished quickly, but is an on-going, lifelong process. There are patients who do achieve and maintain a drug-free existence, and for them the joy of living is great.

References

American Psychiatric Association (1987). *Diagnostic and Statistical Manual of Mental Disorders* (3rd ed. revised). Washington, DC: American Psychiatric Association.

Bennett, G., Vourakis, C., and Woolf, D. S. (Eds.). (1983). *Substance abuse: Pharmacologic, development and clinical perspectives.* New York: John Wiley & Sons, Inc.

Crawford, A. L., and Kilander, V. C. (1980). *Psychiatric nursing: A basic manual.* Philadelphia, F. A. Davis Company.

Delmarest, M. (1981). Cocaine: Middle class high. *Time, 11*(8), 56.

Hollister, L. E. (1985). *Drug tolerance, dependence, and abuse.* Kalamazoo, MI: The Upjohn Company.

Moyer, R. L., and Snider, M. J. (1983). Interpersonal problems of adults. In J. Howe, E. J. Dickason, D. A. Jones, et al. (Eds.), *The handbook of nursing.* New York: John Wiley & Sons, Inc.

Seigfel, R. K (1984). Cocaine smoking disorders: Diagnosis and treatment. *Psychiatric Annals, 14*(10), 728–732.

Smith, D. E., and Wesson, D. R. (1985). *Treating the cocaine abuser.* Center City, MN: Hazelden Foundation.

SECTION FOUR

SPECIAL CONCERNS

Chapter 12

The Patient with Suicidal Ideation

Susan Lewis *William A. McDowell*
Robert J. Gregory

I. STATEMENT OF PURPOSE

When alert to signs of potential or impending suicide and when skilled in intervention, the nurse is often the key person in the prevention of suicide.

The purpose of this chapter is twofold:

- To increase understanding of the underlying aspects of suicidal behavior.
- To provide a framework for nursing care of the patient who is actively or potentially self-destructive.

II. OVERVIEW OF SUICIDAL BEHAVIOR

A. Description of the Problem

Suicide is the physical act of taking one's own life. Almost everyone has experienced the thought of suicide at one point or another, but the individual truly at risk is the individual under stress who possesses inadequate coping skills and few or no support systems.

The potential for suicide may be particularly pronounced in the depressed patient and may also be present in the hyperactive or manic patient when flashes of underlying depression appear. The danger of self-destruction is always great in the agitated patient. With a patient experiencing psychomotor retardation, the danger is most acute with fluctuations into and out of depression; therefore, the period of recovery from depression may be more dangerous than the deepest point of the depression.

There are two types of suicidal patients: the actively suicidal patient and the potentially suicidal patient. The actively suicidal patient attempts suicide frequently. The potentially suicidal patient thinks or talks of death or suicide; he experiences feelings of depression, guilt, helplessness, hopelessness, and worthlessness, and that he lacks a goal in life. He may have a history of suicide attempts. When a potentially suicidal patient is serious in intent, he may at any point become actively suicidal.

Suicide may be planned or committed on impulse. Drugs and/or alcohol may increase suicide potential by lowering inhibitions, decreasing the ability to reason, and increasing impulsive behavior.

B. Incidence

Suicide is considered the tenth leading cause of death and accounts for approximately 25,000 deaths each year (Hackett and Stern 1987). Among college-age populations, suicide is the second or third leading cause of death (Sudak 1982).

Individuals over 60 years of age account for 23% of all suicides. Interestingly, the incidence of suicide among white males rises steadily as age increases, from 13 per 100,000 at age 60 to over 50 per 100,000 at age 85, while the rate of suicide for females and black males increases up to middle age and then declines (Lieff 1984).

The risk of suicide is greater for the patient with a family history of suicide.

Among nonhospitalized individuals, alcohol is a major contributing factor to suicide, and ill health is a significant motive for suicide in both men and women.

The ratio between attempts and completed suicides has been reported as eight to one (Rigdon and Godbey 1984). Males are three to four times more likely to have successful suicide attempts. About 75% of those persons successful in their final attempts had a history of suicide threats or attempts (Campbell 1981). Statistics concerning successful suicides, however, are confusing. Victims often take elaborate precautions to make the death appear natural or accidental and to protect their families from social stigma and facilitate receipt of life insurance. Physicians and coroners may report the death as nonsuicide.

C. Clinical Manifestations

Depression is the most commonly noted psychiatric sign or symptom. Usually, the patient appears sad, with furrowed brow and downcast eyes. He may stare at the floor and make no eye contact with others, or may hide feelings of depression behind a seemingly calm exterior. The patient may or may not express depressive thoughts.

A preoccupation with self and an increasing disinterest in others and the environment may also be noted. The patient may show little interest in personal appearance and grooming, and may dress in dull, colorless, or dark clothing.

Speech and physical movement may be slowed. The patient may speak infrequently and topics of conversation may be limited. The patient usually expresses feelings of helplessness, hopelessness, and worthlessness. The severely depressed patient may not speak at all.

Insomnia is commonly seen, especially during the early morning hours. Disinterest in food, decreased libido, and loss of appetite may occur; however, some patients eat more when depressed. Vague physical complaints such as headaches, heartburn, constipation, fatigue, and weakness may be voiced. The patient may complain of problems with concentration and memory.

Pacing the floor, crying, and wringing of hands may signal an increase in the patient's anxiety. The patient may express fears of insanity. Decreased muscle tone and slumped shoulders may be observed. The content of the patient's conversation may be end-centered, revealing a preoccupation with death-related topics. Reading material may also focus on death. The patient may begin to give away personal possessions. Increased use of drugs and/or alcohol may aggravate the risk of self-harm.

III. NURSING MANAGEMENT

Effective nursing management involves assessment, planning, intervention, and evaluation.

A. Assessment

In the past, it was thought that the patient should never be questioned about suidical thoughts. Today, however, it is recognized that the patient should be questioned carefully about suicidal thinking, planning, and past attempts at suicide in order to make a thorough and accurate assessment of his condition. Questioning the patient about suicidal ideation (self-destructive thoughts) does not "give" him the idea if he hasn't already been considering it. An awareness of the patient's current situation (i.e., degree of depression, psychosis, or intoxication; extent of the feelings of hopelessness, helplessness, and worthlessness; and severity of the illness or emotional crisis) and a knowledge of past suicidal thoughts and attempts are important in the evaluation of suicide potential.

1. Assess the absence or presence of depression. Symptoms include:
   a. Change in weight (loss or gain)
   b. Decreased libido
   c. Depressed mood with sad affect
   d. Diminished performance
   e. Feelings of despair, hopelessness, and worthlessness
   f. Inability to concentrate
   g. Insomnia or other changes in sleeping patterns, especially early morning waking. (Depression is usually more severe in the morning and lessens as the day continues.)
   h. Lack of energy
   i. Loss of appetite
   j. Loss of interest
   k. Poor memory
   l. Withdrawal and isolation from others

   Note: As stated earlier, when the patient is in the depths of depression, he may not have the energy to commit suicide. During the period of recovery, however, as the patient's energy returns, the danger may be much greater. If for no apparent reason a patient who has been severely depressed appears suddenly improved or cheerful, the nurse would be wise to suspect that a decision to commit suicide has been made. The cheerfulness may reflect the sense of relief experienced once a decision has been made.
2. Assess recent losses in the patient's life (i.e., loss of significant other, status, or health) and determine whether or not current grieving is dysfunctional. If the depressed mood interferes with the patient's overall functioning, and severe physical symptoms persist longer than 2 weeks, the depression or grieving is considered dysfunctional and may require treatment.
3. Assess the absence or presence of support systems: Is there anyone available to be with the patient? Are there others in the patient's environment who can provide a source of strength? Is the patient able to reach out to these people for help and support? Conceivably, the nurse and other hospital personnel may be the patient's only support system.

   Note: Suicide risk is greater when the patient has no support systems.
4. Assess the patient's strengths and resources: How has the patient coped with stress and depression in the past? Is the patient able to mobilize resources? Remember, in the very depths of depression the patient may be unable to think clearly, identify alternatives, or make decisions.

5. Assess the absence or presence of psychosis or any other condition that can precipitate impulsive behavior to relieve anxiety:
   a. Extreme fear and anxiety (Rigdon and Godbey 1984).
   b. Hallucinations: Are voices telling the patient that he is no good? Are voices commanding the patient to kill himself and/or others? Tormenting auditory and/or visual hallucinations can precipitate suicide.
   c. Delusional thinking: Delusional thinking that is threatening in content may require close supervision to insure the safety of the patient and others.
   d. The influence of drugs or alcohol.
6. When assessing depressed, agitated, or chronically ill patients, determine both suicidal and homicidal ideation: "Have you had thoughts of taking your life or the life of someone else?"

   The patient may not express his thoughts of suicide unless questioned by the nurse, and it is important to note that many individuals who consider suicide also consider "taking someone with them."
7. When a patient expresses suicidal ideation, assume he is serious until otherwise determined. Suicide threats laced with tones of failure, hopelessness, and self-degradation are the most serious. Threats that are obviously manipulative are less likely to be accomplished but can never be totally disregarded (Lewis et al. 1986). Also remember that the elderly communicate their suicidal intentions less frequently than younger persons (Lieff 1984).
8. Assess the patient's history of suicide attempts: Does the patient have a history of suicide attempts? If so, how many attempts have been made? When were these attempts made? What methods were used?
9. Directly question the patient for a suicide plan: "How did you plan to kill yourself?" or "Have you thought of how you might do it?"

   Assess the lethality of method:
   a. Using a gun, hanging, or jumping from a high place is more lethal and involves greater risk than taking pills or cutting wrists (Rigdon and Godbey 1984), because of the irreversible nature of the former methods.
   b. Assess the availability of means: "Do you now possess a gun? Ammunition? Do you plan to acquire a gun?"
   c. Assess the degree of detail in the plan: "What preparations have you made? Have you chosen a precise time and method?"

B. Planning

Planning of nursing care for the suicidal patient should be based on a comprehensive nursing assessment and subsequent nursing diagnoses. Modification of the nursing care plan should be based on frequently scheduled reassessments of the patient's mental status and evaluation of nursing care.

C. Intervention

1. Prevention

Major factors in the prevention of suicide are an awareness of the signs of potential suicide and a knowledge of what to do when these signs appear. The aware and knowledgeable nurse acts as a liaison between the suicidal patient and those who provide the continuing support and counseling essential to emotional recovery. Indeed, one of the best precautions against suicide is an astute and imaginative nurse who is sensitive to the patient's current and potential behaviors, alert to the possible suicidal methods available to the patient, and accurately aware of the patient's innermost feelings. The depressed patient's life may well depend on the nurse's ability to observe and understand.

The goal of crisis intervention is to persuade the patient to delay his plan to commit suicide. Preventive measures are outlined as follows:

a. Provide understanding: "I understand that you are under extreme stress. Not knowing where to turn, you've decided that suicide is your only alternative."
b. Provide support: "I value you as a fellow human being and I want to help you find other alternatives. It will take some work, but together we can identify those alternative methods for dealing with this stress."
c. Obtain a commitment from the patient: "I want us to make this a joint effort, but a joint effort requires commitment on both of our parts. I want you to contract with me to delay your plans, giving us time to come up with alternative ways of handling your current situation."
d. Reassure the patient: "We will not let you hurt yourself or anyone else."

2. Treatment

a. Psychiatric Hospitalization

In cases of high risk for suicide, psychiatric hospitalization is necessary. The nurse may encourage the patient to seek voluntary admission, but remember that involuntary commitment may be necessary if the individual is actively dangerous to self or others. Commitment procedures vary from state to state and involve legal process through the courts. In most states either family or concerned persons may initiate the procedure. The following information may be helpful:

- The necessary papers must be filed with the county court.
- Document the behavior that proves that involuntary commitment is in the best interest of the patient and those around him, that is, that the patient is a danger to himself and/or others.
- The time period within which officials act on commitment papers varies from state to state.

b. Treatment Team

Once hospitalized, the patient is assigned to a treatment team. The treatment team generally consists of the attending physician, resident physician, psychiatrist, psychiatric nurse consultant, unit nurses, nurses' aides, unit social worker, and any other staff member who is serving as a therapist for the patient. Team members may vary from hospital to hospital.

c. Inpatient Care

The goals of inpatient care are:

- To protect the patient from self-harm until he is able to assume responsibility for himself.
- To meet the physical needs of the patient.
- To establish communication and rapport with the patient.
- To help the patient express feelings of guilt, anger, and hostility rather than keeping these feelings destructively turned inward.
- As the immediate crisis abates, to help the patient identify resources, establish support systems, develop positive coping skills, and participate in psychotherapy.

e. Electroconvulsive therapy

Electroconvulsive therapy (ECT) may be used after the patient has been transferred to a psychiatric facility. ECT can produce dramatic results in the treatment of the severely depressed patient. (See Chapter 1, "The Patient with Depression," for additional information.)

3. Medications

The severely depressed patient may require medication as prescribed by the attending physician. Antidepressant medications such as tricyclics and the monoamine oxidase (MAO) inhibitors are the medications most commonly used for the treatment of depression. (For a detailed discussion of these medications, see Chapter 1, "The Patient with Depression.")

4. Nursing Actions
   a. Define the level of suicidal observation status (SOS). Generally, the attending physician defines the SOS with a written order; however, if the nurse believes a patient is suicidal, she may place the patient on continuous one-to-one observation status pending a physician's evaluation. Three suggested levels of SOS are defined:
      - Level I: Continuous one-to-one observation by an assigned staff member of the patient who exhibits unpredictable and impulsive suicidal behavior and requires very close supervision and continuous, immediate intervention.
      - Level II: Continuous sight observation by a staff person in the area holding the patient who presents a less impulsive risk but still requires close supervision.
      - Level III: For the patient showing improvement, continuous observation is no longer required. Staff observation of the patient at 15-minute intervals often proves sufficient.
   b. A noncompleted suicide attempt, as well as a suicide threat, is an urgent warning. Observe the patient closely at all times and watch for any danger signals. One-to-one observation of the acutely suicidal patient may significantly decrease opportunities for suicide attempts. Observe the patient as he takes medication and watch to make sure that the medication is indeed swallowed. If possible, use liquid medications. Patients may pretend to swallow pills and actually save them for future suicide attempts. It is much easier to be sure the patients have swallowed liquid medication.
   c. Since suicide can be impulsive as well as planned, remove all sharp or dangerous objects from the patient's person and environment. Do not allow the patient to keep cigarette lighters, pocket knives, scissors, metal nail files, glass bottles, or belts and other items that could be used for hanging. Mirrors, equipment, and furniture can also be used for self-harm. The environment should be assessed for such objects, and they should be removed from the patient's room.
   d. Meals may be served on paper service with plastic utensils to decrease the availability of items that could be used for self-harm. Some practitioners believe plastic utensils can also be dangerous and provide a single metal spoon or finger foods only.
   e. Be aware of those times on the ward when the patient is more likely to attempt suicide: early morning hours, Sun-

days, and holidays when the number of on-duty staff is low; visiting hours; and times of increased unit activity, such as mealtime or shift change.

f. To reduce the opportunities for self-destruction and to facilitate close observation, restrict the patient to the unit.
g. When the patient is on Level I observation status and if conditions permit, allow the patient to use the phone or smoking room but only if accompanied by an attendant.
h. To prevent elopement and to maintain a sense of identity with the unit, have the patient dress in pajamas rather than in street clothes.
i. When working with the patient, avoid a gay, overly cheerful approach. This may be interpreted as insensitivity or an uncaring attitude.
j. Offer support against impulses of self-punishment. Tell the patient who is fearful of self-harm, "We will not let you hurt yourself. We will protect you."
k. Do not impose your own feelings or your own view of reality upon the patient. Problems that may seem insignificant to you may be very serious to the patient.
l. Demonstrate respect for the patient. Sincere acceptance and respect can be communicated to even the most deeply depressed patient.
m. Avoid extremes in your own mood when with the patient. Maintaining a consistent attitude will help you be more objective and will encourage the patient to perceive you as accepting and/or respectful.
n. Listen carefully to the patient and find out what is meaningful to him at the moment.
o. Be attentive and show that you care what happens.
p. Listen with sensitivity but remind the patient that suicide is his idea and that other alternatives do exist.
q. To reduce self-centeredness and preoccupation with inward thought and brooding, plan diversional activities in line with the patient's capabilities.
r. Allow the patient to make simple decisions such as what to eat at mealtime and whether or not to watch television. While major decisions made by others may offer the patient much relief, freedom to make these simple decisions provides the patient with a degree of responsibility and some control over his environment.
s. Permit the patient to make suicide threats whenever he feels this need, but
   - Take all statements seriously
   - Do not ignore any threat

- Do not argue about suicide threats with the patient

t. Help the patient to unburden himself; permit him to discuss his innermost feelings. Acknowledge the psychological pain the patient feels without becoming overly sympathetic. Therefore, the nurse will not lose objectivity and thus effectiveness.

u. Continue to evaluate the patient's emotional condition. The nurse's observations are valuable in assessing whether the patient is to remain on or be removed from SOS. Observe and chart:
   - Degree of isolation from others
   - Frequency of crying
   - Degree of eye contact
   - Facial expression
   - Changes in verbalizations. As depression lifts, conversation becomes more hopeful and no longer end-centered. The patient may also be willing to make a "no suicide" contract with staff and may begin to make plans and set goals for the future.
   - Tone of voice—note the presence or absence of inflection. The severely depressed patient may speak in a flat, monotone voice, whereas a patient who is less depressed may speak with greater expressiveness and intonation.
   - Physical stance and position. As the patient becomes less depressed he may sit or stand in a more erect manner, with head up. He may also decrease the physical distance between himself and others.
   - Interest in physical appearance, food, television, family, hobbies, and so on.
   - Level of activity
   - Efforts to socialize

v. Continue to question the patient regarding feelings and plans for self-harm. Determine whether or not major contributing factors—such as intoxication—have been adequately removed or alleviated. Remember that the patient coming out of a severe depression may finally have the energy to make a suicide attempt.

w. Removal from SOS will be effected when the staff physician, in concurrence with the psychiatrist, writes the order.

x. Strenuous exercise such as running or striking motions such as shadowboxing or hitting a punching bag may be of benefit by creating endorphins, which help relieve constipation and increase muscle tone. The patient may also feel a sense of accomplishment, which adds to his sense of well-being.

D. Evaluation/Expected Outcome

Effective nursing management can be evaluated in terms of observable behaviors.

1. The nurse will:
   a. Protect the patient from self-harm until he is able to assume this responsibility for himself.
   b. Meet physical (physiological) needs of the patient until he can do this himself.
2. The patient will:
   a. "Express feelings of guilt, anger and hostility in a constructive manner rather than turning these feelings destructively inward" (Lewis et al. 1986).
   b. Report suicidal ideation, delusions, and/or hallucinations (Rigdon and Godbey 1984).
   c. Report a decreased incidence of suicidal ideation.
   d. Verbalize a desire to live and that he no longer plans to kill himself.
   e. Interact with staff and other patients.
   f. Interact with family and friends.
   g. Formulate alternative coping strategies.
   h. Identify and evaluate situations that precipitate suicidal ideation.
   i. State alternative coping strategies.
   j. Participate with others in unit activities.
   k. Identify and verbalize personal strengths.

E. Evaluation for Referral

When a patient is actively suicidal or at high risk for suicide, it may be difficult to manage the patient on a medical-surgical unit. If medically feasible, it may be wise to transfer the patient to a psychiatric unit, where the physical environment can be more easily controlled. The psychiatric unit is equipped with special windows, doors that may be locked, special furnishings, and facilities for restraining and seclusion if necessary.

IV. POTENTIAL NURSING DIAGNOSES

1. Communication, impaired: verbal, related to
   - low self-esteem
   - impaired thought processes
   - social isolation
2. Coping, ineffective individual, related to
   - disturbances in mood
   - feelings of worthlessness and hopelessness
   - delusions
   - guilt
   - internalized anger
3. Grieving, dysfunctional, related to
   - internalized anger
   - actual or perceived object loss
   - loss of significant others
   - chronic fatal illness
4. Injury, potential for (self-harm), related to
   - suicidal ideation
   - depression
   - internalized anger
5. Powerlessness, related to
   - low self-esteem
   - feelings of hopelessness and worthlessness

V. SUMMARY

Care of the suicidal patient requires an alert, perceptive, and acutely sensitive nurse. It is essential to recognize that the suicidal patient is extremely ill and that good nursing care may make a difference in the life or death of this individual.

References

Campbell, R. J. (1981). *Psychiatric Dictionary* (5th ed.). New York: Oxford University Press.

Hackett, T. P., and Stern, T. A. (1987). Suicide and other disruptive states. In T. P. Hackett and N. H. Cassem (Eds.), *Massachusetts General Hospital handbook of general psychiatry.* Massachusetts: PSG Publishing Co., Inc.

Kim, M. J., McFarland, G. K., and McLane, A. M. (1984). *Pocket guide to nursing diagnoses.* St. Louis: C. V. Mosby Company.

Knowles, R. E. (1984). Anxiety and the affective disorders. In J. Howe, E. J. Dickensen, D. A. Jones, et al. (Eds.), *The handbook of nursing.* New York: John Wiley & Sons.

Lewis, S., McDowell, W. A., and Gregory, R. (1986). Saving the suicidal patient from himself. *RN Magazine* (Dec.), 26–28.

Lieff, J. D. (1984). *Your patient's keeper.* Cambridge, Mass.: Ballinger Publishing Company.

Rigdon, I. S., and Godbey, K. L. (1984). Threats to survival. In J. Howe, E. J. Dickensen, D. A. Jones, et al. (Eds.), *The handbook of nursing.* New York: John Wiley & Sons.

Sudak, H. S. (1982). *Suicide.* Speech delivered at a workshop on management and disturbed behavior, Regional Medical Education Center, Becksville, Ohio.

Taylor, C. M. (1986). *Mereness' essentials of psychiatric nursing* (12th ed.). St. Louis: C. V. Mosby Company.

Veterans Administration (1972). "Suicidal." Section XXVI *Program Guide for Nursing Service.* (G-10, M-2, part V) Washington, DC: Veterans Administration, Department of Medicine and Surgery, pp. 2–60 to 2–62.

Chapter 13

The Patient with Violent Behavior

Eleanor Haven *Vince Piscitello*

I. STATEMENT OF PURPOSE

Although violence is not a diagnosis, managing violent behavior is one of the most difficult problems facing today's nurse. Threats of violence and disruptive behavior are frightening and can occur so rapidly that staff must react with little time for elaborate planning. It is crucial to use a team approach for the prevention and management of violent or disruptive behavior. Safety precautions and methods of intervention should be established and practiced well in advance. This chapter will not address hostage situations, but rather is designed to assist the nurse with the assessment, prevention, and management of violent behavior as it occurs in the day-to-day health care setting.

II. OVERVIEW OF VIOLENT BEHAVIOR

A. Description of the Problem

The violent patient is one whose behavior causes harm to self, others, animals, and/or property. Violence is not a diagnosis, but rather a behavior that can range in intensity from arguing and demanding, to verbal threatening, to physical attack, to brutality and murder.

While a behavioral model would suggest that patients cannot be labelled as "violent" until they have been assaultive or destructive, violent thoughts and verbalizations are common among psychiatric patients and such patients may be considered potentially violent. Nurses are urged to remember that not all violent individuals are mentally ill, and not all violent persons should be treated as patients.

Violence is seen in association with a number of medical and psychiatric conditions. Six diagnostic categories alert the nurse to the potential of violence:

1. *Psychosis*—Patients of concern in this category are primarily manic, rather than schizophrenic. The manic patient's behavior is expansive and entertaining. Staff can forget that this patient is extremely labile and can suddenly become violent.
2. *Personality Disorder*—Patients with antisocial and borderline personality disorders are capable of lashing out wildly with chaotic impulsivity. When frustrated, they may demonstrate extreme rage and be very destructive. Alcohol and drugs further increase their potential for violence.

   Patients with paranoid personality disorders may be of particular concern in the emergency room, where patients are seen quickly. Paranoid patients tend to be vague, aloof, and suspicious, giving limited information. If the nurse is too persistent or too probing in her questioning, these patients may become increasingly anxious and explode into violence.

   See also Chapter 7, "The Patient with an Antisocial Personality Disorder," and Chapter 8, "Patients with Other Personality Disorders."
3. *Brain Dysfunction*—These patients can present with belligerent or violent behavior as a chief complaint. Often they are referred to psychiatry without a thorough medical evaluation. It is crucial to first rule out any physical causes for the behavior. When patients meet one or more of the following criteria, an organic basis for the behavior must be considered:
   a. Disorientation
   b. Changes in affect
   c. Abnormal autonomic signs
   d. Forty years of age or older with no previous history of dementia.

      See also Chapter 6, "The Patient with Brain Dysfunction."
4. *Postictal Confusion and Temporal Lobe Seizure*—Occasionally patients in postictal confusion states can exhibit disruptive or violent behavior. Patients with temporal lobe seizures can also exhibit violence; however, according to the American Psychiatric Association (1974), violence as a direct seizure manifestation is uncommon.
5. *Drug and Alcohol Intoxication*—Intoxicated patients can be belligerent and uncooperative, and can become violent if provoked or frustrated. Patients under the influence of amphetamines or phencyclidine (PCP) can be extremely agitated and violent.

6. *Drug and Alcohol Withdrawal*—Patients with impending delirium tremens (DT's) can be explosive and very difficult to manage. Patients withdrawing from barbiturates can have symptoms similar to those in DT's. Opiate addicts can be dangerous, threatening, and violent when trying to coerce staff into giving them drugs.

   Individuals who are admitted to the hospital go from an independent state to a dependent state, which can be very frightening. This loss of control is many times a precipitating factor in disruptive behavior. Fear, frustration, rejection, inferiority feelings, intrusion into personal space, testing limits, and grief may also contribute to disturbed or violent behavior.

   Violence is time limited, since no one can sustain the energy level necessary for violence over long periods of time. Thus, the patient will exhaust himself in a short time, although it can seem like a very long time to the nurse. This is an important fact for the nurse to keep in mind when managing a violent incident.

B. Incidence

While it has been estimated that less than 5% of psychiatric patients are violent, episodes of violence in society increase every day and health care settings are not exempt.

1. Males aged 15–30 are the highest risk group for violence.
2. Rates of accomplished violence are greater in areas of low socioeconomic status with conditions of dense overcrowding.
3. Cases of homicide and aggravated assault are more prevalent on Friday, Saturday, or Sunday between the evening and early morning hours.
4. Rates of violence are higher among poor, undereducated people having few employment skills.
5. Drugs and alcohol contribute tremendously to rates of accomplished violence because of lowered inhibitions, decreased judgment, and, in some cases, paranoid ideation.
6. Highest risk areas in the health care setting are emergency rooms and admitting areas.
7. People who misuse motor vehicles are responsible for violence in large proportions.

It is difficult to assess the incidence of assaults on health care personnel. Incidents are under-reported because staff fear being blamed.

C. Clinical Manifestations

Violent patients are rarely irrationally or randomly violent, but respond to significant stresses and situations. The victims are usually near and dear ones. The central theme seen in violent behavior is helplessness.

Three clues that alert the nurse to the possibility of violence are: (1) the patient's diagnosis, (2) past history of violence, and (3) present behavior. Behavioral signs that indicate potential for violence include:

1. Excessive motor activity—agitation and pacing, pounding, and slamming
2. Tense posture
3. Grim, defiant affect, clenched teeth
4. Arguing
5. Demanding
6. Clenched fists
7. Talking in a rapid, raised voice
8. Challenging staff
9. Threatening staff

Although it is difficult to predict violence, past history of violence appears to be a fairly reasonable predictor.

III. NURSING MANAGEMENT

A. Assessment

Because prevention is the key issue in the management of disturbed or violent behavior, keen observation and accurate assessment are critical factors. Nurses who are empathetic, sincere, and observant will often have an advantage, although this does not assure safety because the process may have escalated to a critical point before the nurse interacts with the patient. For example, if the nurse can take measures to help the patient feel less helpless and more in control, he may calm down. Giving space and acknowledging his anger and frustration may defuse some of the anger. Telling the patient "We won't let you hurt yourself or anyone else" may be reassuring.

Initial assessments may have to be made rapidly if a situation is approaching or has reached a dangerous stage. More thorough assessment should follow when things are under control. Three major areas are considered in the assessment of disruptive or violent behavior: patient, self, and environment.

1. Patient

Knowledge of the patient is an advantage in assessment of his behavior. Know the patient's history, diagnosis, and treatment, and observe his general behavior. Nurses who float or are employed part-time sometimes find themselves at greater risk than full-time, permanent nurses who have the advantage of knowing the patients on a daily basis.

a. Question for a history of violent behavior—history of assault, destructive episodes, spouse abuse, child abuse, reckless driving, destruction of property, and prior suicide attempts.
b. Suicidal patients should be questioned for homicidal urges. Sometimes a patient who intends to kill himself plans to take someone with him.
c. Question for a criminal history and previous arrests for violence.
d. Assess the nature of present threats, whether indirect or direct. Indirect—"I'm afraid I may lose control and hurt someone." Direct—"I'm going to kill everyone in this clinic, starting with you."
e. Question the patient frankly and honestly for details. Whom does he want to hurt? What are his reasons? How much has he been thinking about violence? Has he made any definite plans? What is the most violent thing he has ever done? Is the method lethal?
f. Evaluate the ability of the patient to translate anger and agitation into action. How likely is he to carry out threats? What are his inner controls? For example, the nurse may ask the patient, "On a scale from one to ten, with one being not likely and ten being very likely—where are you?" (Psychiatric personnel have a duty to warn the patient's intended victims. This should be done within the guidelines of the agency. See Chapter 21, "Legal Issues in Psychiatry," p. 293.)
g. Assess the history of temper tantrums, setting fires, and cruelty to animals when the patient was a child. These are clues that someone is likely to be violent as an adult.
h. Assess for recent personal or economic loss, such as the death of a loved one or the loss of a job or income.
i. Assess for a past history of head trauma and/or seizures.
j. Assess for the presence of hallucinations commanding the patient to hurt himself or others.
k. Assess for delusions. Be cautious when delusional patients have fantasies of violence. For example, "You are trying to poison me!" or "This place is a Vietcong prison camp." A patient may believe he is God's Avenging Angel.
l. Determine whether the patient is carrying any weapons or has access to weapons.
m. Examine school behavior, military history, and driving history.

n. Assess social and cultural factors that may contribute to violence.
o. Observe nonverbal behaviors:
   - Presence of anxiety
   - Tense or angry facial expression
   - Extreme fluctuation in mood
   - Agitation and excess motor activity
   - Startle response
   - Tense, rigid posture
   - Loud voice with pressured speech
p. If the patient ceases his anxious behavior and suddenly switches to a tense, uneasy stillness, this is an indication of danger.
q. Search the patient for weapons on his person and in his belongings before admission to the hospital. Even if the patient is willing to give up the weapon, do not take it directly from him. Have the patient place the weapon on the floor and scoot it out of reach. Security guards should be called to take charge of the weapon and sometimes to assist with the search of the patient. Security should be notified if a patient refuses to give up a weapon.

2. Self

It is important for the nurse to assess herself and her personal feelings about the patient, the work environment, and events occurring externally or in other relationships that may be a hinderance to the therapeutic relationship. The nurse must be aware of her own activities, moods, and reactions, since victims can sometimes precipitate or provoke violence. Tone of voice communicates the speaker's attitude far more accurately than the words spoken. Body language is important. A nurse who stands a little to the side of the patient and with her arms at her sides communicates openness and acceptance. A nurse who stands with arms crossed, has a tense posture, and makes intense eye contact may communicate a threat.

The nurse must rely on her "gut reaction" to a situation. An uneasy feeling while listening to a disturbed patient can be a valuable indication of the potential for violence.

3. Environment

The nurse must assess the environment, keeping in mind that when patients enter the health care setting, they are looking for a secure, stable environment. An environment that gives the appearance of being cold or chaotic increases the risk of violence. The patient is quick to observe problems in the environment such as disorganization, staff personality clashes, and disgruntled staff. It is important for team building and cohesiveness to be an integral part of the staff development program, thereby placing the environment at low risk.

a. Assess the presence and availability of staff to assist in an emergency.
b. Assess items in the environment that could be used as weapons—IV poles, glass bottles, sharp instruments, cue sticks, and the like.
c. Assess items in the environment that could be used for protection—desks, beds, chairs, and so on.
d. Know how to summon help.

B. Planning

The planning of nursing care for the violent patient should be based on the aforementioned risk assessment and analysis. The nursing care plan should encompass a nursing diagnosis that reflects the level of risk and should change as the risk increases or decreases.

A hospital plan for the prevention and management of disruptive behavior should be developed well ahead of time, just like the fire safety plan. Good organization and team building strategies are key measures in prevention and control. Staff should be given training in verbal and physical management techniques with periodic reviews. Thus, when an incident occurs, staff intervention will be within specific established guidelines. Staff will know what to do, and safety for the patient and staff will be facilitated.

C. Intervention

1. Prevention

As previously emphasized, prevention is the primary consideration in the management of disturbed behavior. The nurse who is alert to signs of mounting tension can intervene before a situation escalates to violence. A number of simple and prudent measures can deter violence.

a. Verbal techniques are critical in preventing violent behavior. Used with an empathetic manner that conveys calmness, control, and willingness to help, verbal techniques are extremely effective. Remember, feelings of helplessness, fear of losing control, and/or psychosis are very painful, and the patient wants relief. If the nurse can convey her willingness to provide relief, 85%–90% of patients will respond to verbal intervention (Dubin et al. 1981).
b. Commonsense measures can promote safety:
   - Do not be complacent or think violence can't occur.
   - Do not allow a potentially violent patient to get between the nurse and the door.

- Know where other staff members are at all times.
- Long hair, neckties, dangling earrings, and scarves create a greater hazard risk for injury in a violent situation.
- Doors to seclusion rooms should open outward to prevent patient from barricading himself and/or staff in the room.
- Patients with a history of violence who are suspected of being dangerous should be interviewed in a quiet area. Noise and confusion can increase agitation.
- When in doubt, have security stand by (out of sight, if necessary).
- In an office, the desk should be situated so that the nurse cannot become trapped in the room.
- With a suspicious or paranoid patient, giving a few options may decrease his fear.
- Leaving the door to the office open may increase the comfort of the patient and the nurse.
- Offering food and drink to the patient is very soothing. It conveys concern and can decrease tension and anxiety. With an unknown patient or one who is extremely agitated, it is best to offer cold beverages.
- The nurse should never interview a potentially violent patient without letting other staff know where she will be and arranging to have other staff check on her every few minutes.
- Stand at least a leg's length away from the patient.
- Do not turn your back to the patient.
- Flag the chart and treatment plan to alert other staff to a potentially violent patient.

c. Private offices or isolated areas should have alarm systems for summoning help. The system should be tested and situations role-played by staff ahead of time to reduce the risk of harm through failure of the system.

d. Some health care facilities have metal detectors because of the increasing number of weapons being brought into hospitals and clinics.

e. Because of changes in the health care system for third-party reimbursement (diagnostic related groupings [DRG's]) and in utilization review, nursing homes are seeing changes in their patient population; thus many nursing homes are offering classes in the prevention and management of dangerous behavior.

f. Every health care setting should have policies and procedures for the prevention and management of violent behavior. All staff should be oriented to these policies and procedures, and should attend regularly scheduled refresher courses. Security staff should be included in the training. This will help ensure the competency of all employees involved in managing an incident.

g. A committee should be formed to review all incidents that occur. Members should be multidisciplinary. Incidents should be reviewed for fact-finding, *NOT* fault-finding. Individuals involved in acts of violence are more likely to be candid when assigning blame is not the focus of the review. A review should include the time of day, staffing patterns, environmental conditions, and condition of the patient at the time of the incident; current hospital policies and procedures; and interventions used for control of the violent situation.

2. Treatment

Several treatment measures are used with violent or potentially violent patients.

a. *Verbal intervention*—Verbal techniques are utilized as the primary mode of intervention and are effective in the majority of cases. It is essential to treat the patient with respect and as a human being. Communication with the patient should continue throughout the entire process of dealing with the patient, even if physical intervention is required. Often allowing the patient to express his feelings and acknowledging his right to them will defuse a situation.
b. *Chemical restraint*—Medication can be very effective with the disturbed, agitated patient. (Medications are in the next section of this chapter).
c. *Physical intervention*—Physical management techniques are sometimes necessary when other methods are not sufficient to prevent a patient who is out of control from harming himself or others. These techniques should be used only when there is no other alternative. No matter how skilled staff may be in the use of physical management techniques, there is always a risk of injury to the patient or the staff when "hands on" techniques are required.

Some nursing management courses promote unrealistic expectations in the nursing staff, which only puts them at greater risk of being injured. Nurses need to be aware that they are not superhuman, even though they've "had the course."

Personnel who attend courses on managing violent behavior should take the information seriously, keeping in mind that it is every health care worker's responsibility. In many hospitals violent behavior is considered only the nursing staff's responsibility, so that when an episode occurs, other health care professionals suddenly disappear.

d. *Restraints and seclusion*—Restraints and seclusion are a last resort and should be thought of not as an end, but as the beginning of an intervention.
   - Leather restraints are used to restrict the patient's movement in order to protect himself or others from harm. Some patients even request to be put in restraints when they fear losing control.
   - The seclusion room offers the opportunity to master a small space and decrease sensory stimuli, thereby providing relief. Seclusion provides a "time-out" in a safe environment.
   - Close observation and planning for the return of the patient to his unit is critical in preventing recurring incidents.

     Criteria for the nursing care of patients in restraints or seclusion should be part of the policies and procedures of every health care facility.

     Careful monitoring of the patient is critical because of the danger to him when he is in restraints or seclusion. He is in a totally dependent state. Frequent observation and documentation is a must during this time. Skin care, hydration, nutrition, personal hygiene, and toileting must be part of the nursing care plan. Specific procedures should be developed by each hospital outlining how these services will be provided and their frequency. The patient should be viewed as needing intensive care, that is, one-to-one nursing care. While the patient is in restraints or seclusion, questions should be raised as to what brought about the incident. What might have to change to prevent it from recurring?

     Communicating with the patient while he is in restraints or seclusion prevents isolation and lets him know that this is not punitive intervention but a therapeutic one. All staff who assisted placing the patient in restraints or seclusion should visit the patient, thus allowing the patient to know there are no hard feelings and everyone is sensitive to what happened.

e. *Alternative interventions*—Using alternative interventions can be helpful in calming the patient. Some suggested interventions include:
   - Relaxation exercises
   - Walking or other physical exercise
   - Cigarettes and/or coffee

- Listening to music
- Use of a quiet room

3. Medications

Medication can provide welcome relief for the agitated and anxious patient when the reasons for medication are explained to him. If a PRN medication order is available, it should be offered to the patient early, before he escalates to the point where he is more likely to refuse it. Ask the patient, "Would you like something to help calm you?" It should be kept in mind that what the patient is going through is a very unpleasant state.

Rapid tranquilization of the acutely ill psychotic patient can be extremely effective. Some agencies prefer oral concentrate and some prefer the use of intramuscular injections.

Haloperidol (Haldol) can be given in 5–10 mg doses IM every ½ hour up to a total of 40–60 mg/day.

Thiothixene (Navane) can be given 10–15 mg of oral concentrate or 10 mg IM every ½ hour depending on the age, weight, and physical condition of the patient. Vital signs should be taken prior to each dose. Ordinarily, 1–3 doses are sufficient (Dubin et al. 1981).

If sedation is needed, medications such as thioridazine (Mellaril), chlorpromazine (Thorazine), or mesoridazine (Serentil) can be used (Dubin et al. 1981).

Sometimes the nurse is faced with an acutely ill psychotic patient who refuses medication altogether. In many states medication can be given if the situation is an emergency; however, the nurse should be aware of the laws of her state and the policy of her hospital that govern these instances.

4. Nursing Actions

Assessment of a patient's level of anxiety is essential to making the appropriate choice for therapeutic intervention. As stated earlier, violence does not occur in a vacuum, but is a component part of a four-level process (see Table 13–1).

Phase I intervention should be supportive, empathetic listening skills that are easily perceived as genuine. Phase II intervention should be supportive, with the addition of limit setting. Staff must not set limits that they are not prepared to

Table 13–1. FOUR LEVELS OF TENSION AND THE APPROPRIATE INTERVENTION

Patient	Staff
I. Basic anxiety	Verbal support
II. Threatening	Limit setting
III. Acting-out	Team approach (PCS)
IV. Anxiety reduction	Therapeutic rapport—verbal support

enforce. Phase III intervention makes use of the team approach (personal contact skills, or PCS). Phase IV intervention involves empathetic listening, with a therapeutic rapport evolving from the emotional flooding following the crisis situation.

a. Supportive verbal intervention
   - Listen empathetically with a posture of calmness and control. This can be difficult to master because the nurse may feel threatened and envision an ensuing danger.
   - Convey a genuine concern for the patient's situation. This will reduce anxiety and promote further communication in most cases. When the nurse is perceived as a truly caring person, and not one who is merely providing "therapeutic lip service" and rhetoric, the patient is more likely to comply with requests.
   - Speak softly so that the patient will have to lower his voice in order to hear.
   - Body language should be consistent with what is being said.
   - Allow the patient to verbalize his anger. Acknowledging his anger may sometimes defuse the situation.
   - Don't argue with the patient.
   - Don't attempt to reason with a patient whose behavior is out of control.
   - Don't show fear.
   - Don't make promises that can't be fulfilled.
   - Don't make threats or imply that the patient will be punished for his anger.
   - Show respect for the pateint as a human being.
   - Utilize any staff member who has good rapport with the patient. This may not necessarily be the nurse or physician, but may be a nurse's aide or someone from housekeeping or dietary.
   - Threats to harm self or others should be taken seriously.
   - Do not crowd or touch the patient. Note his use of "body space." Potentially violent patients have a body buffer zone that is greater than normal. This zone is the area that he defends against intrusion from others. A patient who moves back and forth from an approaching nurse may feel crowded and be more prone to violence. He will guard his back and be wary of sudden approaches.

b. Limit Setting

   If the patient's anxiety continues to mount, he will move to the next level of tension—the threatening phase. This is characterized by statements such as, "Go to hell!" "I don't have to listen to you!" or "If I don't see a doctor right now, someone will be very sorry!" Often the nurse sees a clenched fist and a very angry facial expression. She will feel her own anxiety mount as she perceives an approaching danger. The appropriate intervention at this point is to remain verbally supportive, but to add a directive, limit-setting component to the intervention.

Limit setting does not imply threatening the patient in hopes that he will back down, but rather involves setting appropriate limits to contain the situation. The key to successful limit setting is setting only those limits that are enforceable. Once a limit is set, for example, "Let's go into the conference room and talk," and the patient says, "I'm not going anywhere with you," staff must either be prepared to escort a person who is ready to act-out or do nothing. Doing nothing is a signal that staff are helpless to assist the patient in gaining control. This can be frightening to the patient, causing futher escalation and loss of control. Depending on the situation, the nurse may make a *request* ("Please put the chair down") or give a *command* ("Put the chair down") but never issue a threat.

c. Team approach (personal contact skills)

Certain patients do not respond to verbal intervention no matter how skilled the team is in these techniques. As threats approach the acting-out phase, physical intervention may be required to contain the patient. A team approach is mandatory. No staff member should attempt to subdue a patient without assistance.

The physical approach advocated is the personal contact skills (PCS) approach. In order to learn PCS techniques, one must be taught by competent instructors in a formal training session which allows for hands-on role-play and practice of skills that involve take-down and immobilization of the patient. The following seven rules are important for personal contact skills to be successful in containing the patient:

- Recognize mounting tension.
- In situations of potential violence, other patients and visitors should be removed to a calm, nonstimulating area. If the nurse is alone, she must consider her personal safety and not place herself at higher risk. For example, she should not take a potentially violent patient to an area where she cannot be observed by other staff members.
- Do not enlist the aid of other patients in an intervention.

- Approach the patient with a calm, matter-of-fact, and reasonable manner.
- Protect the patient from injury during an intervention.
- Staff who have been trained and are skilled in physical intervention techniques should be readily available to assist in a crisis situation.
- Continue to talk with the patient throughout the intervention.

A closer look at the techniques of PCS is in order. Most physical techniques used to control acting-out behavior emphasize a quick means of gaining control. This may involve a serious struggle for control while the individual is at his highest energy level; such a struggle can be dangerous and team efforts may be thwarted. Other techniques are based on a "show of force" where every available staff member lines up against one angry person. If the patient does not back down, the whole "wall" converges and grabs out, creating a melee where the potential of injury to patient and/or staff is very real.

The PCS approach, however, suggests the use of a three-person team. The nurse who initially became involved with the patient or the person who has the best chance of defusing the situation becomes the impromptu team leader. A brief meeting to create a plan of action is held that includes anxiety level assessment, intervention to begin with, and code phrases for the "hands-on" intervention of Phase III (e.g., "Mr. Jones, I want you to SIT IN THE BROWN CHAIR": "sit in the brown chair" signals the team to use hands-on techniques).

Once this plan of action has been discussed and understood by all team members, the team leader should approach the patient in a calm, supportive manner. The approach should be effected at a 90-degree angle to the patient, rather than in a face-to-facc manner; such an approach is perceived as a lesser threat by the patient. The team should be prepared to set enforceable limits if the patient escalates to the threatening phase. Enforcement should be with the minimum amount of force necessary; they may simply escort the patient to the "brown chair" while remaining alert for the possibility of a struggle.

If a physical struggle should occur, the team would use the PCS approach to contain the crisis while giving the patient verbal cues that it is okay to stop struggling. Often, an individual believes that if the struggle has begun it is necessary to carry it through to the end. By giving the patient permission to quit, the individual knows the nurse is not angry but is concerned for his safety.

Using a wrong intervention, or not being prepared to use an appropriate intervention, can be dangerous to both the patient and staff. For example, if the patient has escalated to the threatening phase (e.g., "If I don't get Valium right now, I'll punch you out"), but the staff is continuing to use the supportive approach without setting limits (e.g., "Mr. Jones, you seem upset; would you like to sit down and talk about it?"), a crisis may be precipitated. It is important to set limits at the appropriate time (e.g., "Mr. Jones, when you talk like that it scares me and I can't be of much help to you when I'm scared, so please lower your voice and let's sit down and discuss your situation"), remembering that staff must be prepared to enforce these limits if necessary; thus the PCS team must be available and alerted to the situation.

The confidence and control of a well-trained team will most likely be perceived by the patient who is losing control and will provide him with a feeling of safety. An example is the black belt in karate: this individual rarely gets into fights because of his ability to demonstrate confidence and control; an aggressor quickly perceives this control, and the need for escalating threats to get the opponent to back down are not necessary. The aggressor feels the expert is capable of handling whatever situation arises, and takes the advice of the expert to calm down.

d. Therapeutic rapport/verbal support

Once a patient is physically in control, an interesting phenomenon occurs. This is Phase IV, or the anxiety-reduction phase. The patient usually begins to flood the nurse with insight as to the underlying causes for his behavior, and a therapeutic rapport may be established. If intervention was handled professionally, a positive rapport should evolve. If the intervention was handled inappropriately, using excessive physical force, an atmosphere of mistrust may ensue.

e. Documentation

After a crisis situation has occurred, documentation is critical. This should be done as soon as possible after the incident. Details of the incident should be explained; note the type of intervention used and the reasons for this choice.

D. Evaluation/Expected Outcomes

1. The nurse will:
   a. Provide a safe environment for the patient and others.
   b. Protect the patient and others from self-harm or acting-out of violent and destructive impulses until the patient can assume responsibility for himself.
   c. Help the patient express feelings of rage and hostility in a constructive, safe, and acceptable manner.
   d. Provide acceptance.
   e. Discuss with other staff any incidents that occur. Allow staff to express their feelings and evaluate how the situation was handled, without assigning blame.

2. The patient will:
   a. "Regain" control of his behavior.
   b. Recognize the problems he creates with his behavior.
   c. Understand his feelings of anger and hostility.
   d. Learn to cope with anger and hostility in ways that do not harm himself or others.
   e. Identify factors that elicit feelings of helplessness and threats to the "self."
   f. Identify consequences of his behavior.
   g. Seek help before losing control.

E. Evaluation for Referral

Documentation is the major component in evaluation for referral. The key issues to be documented are:

1. Patient's positive and negative behaviors
2. Intervention that was successful in assisting the patient to change negative behaviors:
   a. Verbal
   b. Medication
   c. Physical
3. Any alternative interventions that were used
4. The patient's support system
5. Nursing diagnosis
6. Other major diagnosis—and the drugs the patient is taking

IV. POTENTIAL NURSING DIAGNOSES

1. Aggressive coping mode, related to
   - anger
   - hostility
   - feelings of helplessness
   - impulsivity
   - impaired judgment
   - impaired thought processes
2. Anxiety, related to
   - perceived threats
   - fear of loss of control
   - restlessness and agitation

3. Coping, ineffective individual, related to
   - delusions
   - hallucinations
   - dependency needs
   - low self-esteem
4. Decision-making, impaired/ineffective, related to
   - poor insight
   - impaired judgment
   - feelings of worthlessness
   - impaired thought processes
5. Fear, related to
   - feelings of helplessness
   - delusions
   - hallucinations
   - anger
   - hostility
6. Grieving, dysfunctional, related to
   - perceived or actual loss
   - internalized anger
   - inadequate coping skills
7. Injury, potential for, related to
   - poor impulse control
   - verbal aggression or abuse of others
   - hostility
   - belligerence
   - denial and projection
8. Thought processes, alterations in, related to
   - thought disturbances
   - delusions
   - hallucinations
9. Violence (other-directed), potential, related to
   - anger
   - hostility
   - feelings of helplessness
   - denial
   - projection
   - poor impulse control
10. Violence (self-directed), potential for, related to
   - suicidal ideation
   - poor impulse control
   - poor self-esteem

V. SUMMARY

Nursing personnel often have the primary responsibility for handling disorderly or violent patients because of their closeness and intensity of contact. Care of patients who have a potential for violence requires the nurse to be sensitive, empathetic, observant, calm, and caring.

Nurses must talk openly about the possibility of violence and assist other members of the team in dealing with it, should a situation occur. In-service training with role-playing can make a vital difference. One must alway keep in mind that there is no guarantee against violence, but courses on managing violence can reduce the number of incidents and the severity of injuries when a violent incident occurs.

References

American Psychiatric Association (1974). *Clinical aspects of the violent individual.* Washington, DC: American Psychiatric Association.

Dubin, W. R., Benfield, T., and Berger, M. M. (1981). Management of violent patients. A program excerpted from *Management of Violent Patients in the Community,* a symposium presented by the Department of Education and Training, South Beach Psychiatric Center, New York City, NY. Sponsored by Roerig, a division of Pfizer Pharmaceuticals, New York.

Veterans Administration Southeastern Regional Medical Education Center (1987). *The Prevention and Management of Disruptive Behavior,* a course presented by SERMEC, Birmingham, AL.

Chapter 14

The Patient with Sexual Problems or Differences

Robert J. Gregory *Susan Lewis*
William A. McDowell

I. STATEMENT OF PURPOSE

When knowledgeable about sexuality, and aware of taboos, myths, and confusion surrounding the topic, the nurse is capable of acting effectively with patients having problems relating to sexuality. The nurse can recommend and manage many needed interventions, provide helpful counseling and education, promote treatment, and refer a patient to appropriate programs.

This chapter is designed for use by the nurse to:

- Increase understanding of the patient with problems that involve sexuality.
- Facilitate nursing management by describing steps that can be taken to minimize problems and to provide care needed for the patient.

II. OVERVIEW OF SEXUAL PROBLEMS OR DIFFERENCES

A. Description of the Problem

A sexual problem can be physical, psychological, social, and/or legal. A sexual difference can be physical, psychological, or social, and can lead to many psychological, moral, legal, and social complications. Sexuality is pervasive, affecting all human beings from the beginning to the end of life. Problems for patients develop and emerge in many ways in various settings and contexts. Some areas of special interest to the nurse include crisis intervention, education to prevent problems, counseling and advising, treatment, and referral to specialized programs.

Broad categories of patients may include at least the following: victims (survivors) of rape, incest, or other related trauma; homosexuals; those who have a sex-change operation; those who undergo a major physical change such as spinal cord injury or cardiac patients; seductive, sexually aggressive, or flagrant sexually acting-out patients; those who attend sex education classes; persons seeking help at contraception clinics; patients with sexually transmitted disease (such as chlamydia, herpes, or human immunodeficiency virus [HIV] infection); couples who are unsuccessful in achieving pregnancy; women and their partners who are contemplating or undergoing abortion; patients considering a penile implant; and persons unable to accomplish the sexual act with satisfaction to self and a partner. Deviant sexual behavior is largely in the eye of the beholder, but certain acts are regarded as offensive to various groups of people and bring about social sanctions, enmity, and even violence against the perpetrator(s). Frequently, moral and legal complications add to the physical, psychological, and social problems that may exist (Clinard and Meir 1975).

Sexuality is an inherent aspect of every human being. The physiological act of intercourse and resulting reproduction is but a small part of engagement in sexual behavior. Our social mores have made and continue to make sexuality a taboo topic that is difficult for some patients and medical personnel to address. If a nurse is secure in her own sexuality, knowledgeable about the anatomical and physiological aspects of sex, and able to converse using words capable of being understood by the patient, then a great deal of work can be accomplished. However, until the patient and the nurse develop the rapport and trust sufficient to talk about problems relating to sexuality, little can be achieved in nursing practice and treatment. Many clinicians feel inadequate or uncomfortable discussing or confronting the patient with problems of sexuality and therefore avoid this aspect of care altogether (Haber et al. 1978). In these cases, patients can be referred to clinicians with special training in treating sexual problems.

There are many highly trained, well-qualified professionals, and these people and their programs constitute valuable resources. Referral to such resources should be undertaken when and as appropriate, for there are limits to the assistance that can be offered by the nurse (Masters and Johnson 1966, 1970; Kaplan 1979; Kilmann and Mills 1983).

B. Incidence

Sexual problems may lead to various forms of destructive behavior that affect the comfort and security of others. In one sense, nearly everyone is subject to sexual problems at some point in life (Kinsey et al. 1948, 1953; Masters and Johnson 1966, 1970). Many individuals have emotional "scars" from initial sexual experiences and the learning process involved in social interaction that leads to intimacy. In another sense, the manifestation of sexual problems seen by the medical profession is extremely limited in number. In large part, the ability of the nurse to identify, discuss, and work with patients on matters of sexuality will determine the incidence of the problem. Greater sensitivity, skill in eliciting information, and interest can facilitate identification, analysis, evaluation, and resolution of problems.

C. Clinical Manifestations

1. General

As patients present in psychiatric or other settings, the nurse will have many opportunities to observe and consider whether to explore or intervene in issues related to sexuality. Some of the potential indicators worthy of being studied include some of the following areas.

There are *developmental stages* at which particular patterns of sexual problems may emerge. For example, adolescence is associated with the learning process during which exploration and growth take place. Events that may occur during this time include unwanted pregnancies, transmission of venereal disease, and rape, as well as learning of sexual roles, methods of building relationships, and achievement of sexual satisfaction.

There are *physical factors* involved that can lead to serious problems, including HIV infection and various other sexually transmitted diseases. Specific medical syndromes or diagnostic categories may be indicative of needs.

There are *responses to trauma* that may inherently include sexuality. A person with a spinal cord lesion or a myocardial infarction will have many questions and concerns about future sexual roles and options. A person who was raped or sexually traumatized will have grief and emotional reactions that can be worked through so that residual guilt, suffering, and emotional devastation are minimized.

There are *social groupings* who regard sexuality differently than do others, and the consequent differences may lead to sexual problems (the gay community, for example). These people may attract attention because of differences that are not necessarily problems for them. Members of the gay community, as well as persons who have unusual fetishes or patterns of behavior, may be self-identified or be singled out by members of the community and treated in significantly different ways. In a hospital setting, these patients can generally be regarded as would any other person, but the nurse must be aware that some patients, staff, or members of the public may have hostile reactions if sexual differences are known. Persons who undergo a sex change operation may attract unusual interest by members of the public and/or media. Many other matters such as abortion, nudity, or bestiality may elicit violent reactions by members of the public.

There are *specific individuals variously identified as violent, seductive, aggressive,* and so on, who may be receiving nursing care for other reasons. For example, accused rapists may attract a great deal of community attention. In prisons, these men are frequently regarded as being at the bottom of the "pecking order" and are subjected to harassment or assaults.

At times, certain psychiatric patients may display inappropriate sexual behavior on the ward or may behave seductively to staff. The nurse must address these situations in a therapeutic and nonjudgmental but firm manner.

There are *programs* dealing with matters relating to sexuality that are offered by contraception clinics, sex therapy programs, fertility clinics, and sexually transmitted disease clinics, and, more recently, programs designed to teach, improve, or enhance sexual skills and performance. Nurses may engage in educational programs to inform individuals and groups in the community about various aspects of sexuality, including prevention of disorders (Qualls et al. 1978). The nursing role in these programs may be highly specialized.

2. Specific

   Characteristics and symptoms of patients who have sexual problems *may* include the following:

   a. Directly or indirectly reporting sexual trauma or problems
   b. Being insecure, fearful, and resentful in attitude and behavior towards members of the opposite sex
   c. Exhibiting reported hostile and rebellious behavior toward others
   d. Having feelings of self-pity, depression, guilt, helplessness, and hopelessness
   e. Having feelings of loneliness, isolation, and being unloved, without the ability or skills to engage and interact successfully with others
   f. Lacking in self-respect and related promiscuity

g. Being hedonistic with low tolerance for pain (emotional and physical) and frustration
h. Having a seductive or overly likeable and charming personality
i. Possessing the uncanny ability to break rules
j. Being adept at maneuvering other persons into the position of being "guilty"

III. NURSING MANAGEMENT

Effective nursing management involves assessment, short- and long-term planning, intervention during acute phases and over long-term convalescence, and evaluation. In managing the treatment of persons with sexual differences, the authors recommend 5 P's: Protection of Other People and Patients from Harassment; Positive and Active Intervention; Programs in the Community; Prevention through Education; and Practical Planning.

Protection of Other People and Patients from Harassment

Protection of other people and other patients from harassment by the patient is crucial to treatment. People have a right to security and freedom from harassment or unwanted sexual advances. The patient with sexual problems has no right to infringe on the rights and security of other persons. Also, the patient with sexual problems cannot obtain appropriate treatment or counseling from other patients or from staff members who do not have specialized training in these areas. The nurse must be aware that some individuals do agress sexually against others and that such irresponsible behavior should be prevented as much as possible through appropriate nursing planning and actions (Qualls et al. 1978, Chap. 4).

Positive and Active Intervention

Positive and active intervention by the nurse is crucial. A passive, wait-and-see approach will practically guarantee that nothing happens in the way of initiation of discussion about sexuality or treatment. The nurse should assure that rapport with patients is developed, that situations are then set up during which there is appropriate privacy and opportunity to talk, and that leading questions are asked to open and develop a discussion. Neglect of the topic is too frequently the case, and the tendency to avoid such discussions will block any short- or long-term changes.

Programs in the Community

There are individuals and professionals who can be helpful, and other resources that can be called upon, for specific needs and situations. The nurse should be well acquainted with these various resources in the community and have a working knowledge of them. Being able to refer patients to particular programs constitutes a most important and valuable intervention. Contrary to some beliefs and expectations, there are well-trained and competent therapists who can assist patients or clients in resolving problems relating to sexuality with an excellent degree of success.

Prevention through Education

Prevention of sexual problems through education is essential to develop an appropriate individual program for a patient as well as to teach people in various settings (Qualls et al. 1978). Steps that can be taken by a nurse to promote prevention through education include:

1. Be knowledgeable about anatomy and physiology, particularly of the genitourinary and reproductive systems. Also be aware of the larger context of human relationships, including psychological and social aspects.
2. Learn and be able to use both technical and slang vocabularies in discussions about sexuality.
3. Be secure in your own being and personhood as well as in the role of nurse.
4. Know and be able to call upon appropriate community resources and helpful professionals and people.
5. Become desensitized to words or concepts that "trigger" strong emotions or negative feelings. Be aware of how trigger words may affect other people and yourself.
6. Become an exceptionally good listener so that you can "read between the lines" and be aware of your own reactions and responses as you listen.
7. Be aware of the needs for privacy and "alone" time required to work through grief, loss, and trauma.
8. Be aware that some persons have needs and take actions to exploit, express hostility, and otherwise manifest their own

inner turmoil in harmful ways to others. Be aware that a colleague can be invited to work with you and your patient in risky situations. Sex therapy programs often use two therapists, one male and one female, and nurses can set up counseling or other interventions in the same way.

9. Intervention techniques may vary in their effectiveness with patients at different times and in different settings. Be able to intervene in more than one style, depending largely upon needs of the patient.
10. Calm, matter of fact, business-like attitudes and behaviors may be conducive to treatment of some people whose lives are in turmoil or who have been going through an agonizing period. Warmth and cheerfulness may be useful to others. Understand and learn to modify your own attitudes and behaviors to be able to present the most important attributes needed by the patient. Similarly, be aware of your values about sexuality and, while respecting those values, listen to and learn about the values held by the patient. Govern treatment by the needs of the patient, not by your own values alone.
11. Small groups may be helpful; learn to use the dynamics of small groups as a tool in therapeutic work. This can include family and peers.
12. Be especially aware of labels and classifications, since they jeopardize any real human contact. Individual differences are likely to be the rule, even though the labels attached are similar.

Practical Planning

The nurse can work with individuals in specific ways to promote healthy attitudes and behaviors in matters relating to sexuality. Not only can particular problems be successfully treated, but skills and competence in sexuality can also be enhanced (D'Augelli and D'Augelli 1985; Sarrel and Sarrel 1979; LoPiccolo and Miller 1975). The nurse can assist individual patients to accomplish the following steps:

1. Develop an appropriate and positive body image
2. Overcome guilt, shame, and inhibitions
3. Recognize and be able to discuss with a partner those behaviors that are fulfulling and satisfying
4. Reduce conflict and confusion about sexuality and sex roles
5. Attain self-confidence, ability, and skills in a sexual relationship

A. Assessment

1. Sexual abuse, trauma and crisis
   a. Identify the incident that occurred—date, time, and details
   b. Note the patient's overall appearance and any evidence of physical trauma—bruises, internal and external; vaginal and/or anal bleeding and lacerations
   c. Note any hygiene measures the patient has taken following the incident—for example, bathing, douching, or cleansing of wounds
   d. Conduct a physical exam including vaginal, anal, and/or oral assessment
   e. Collect any necessary specimens—semen; dried secretions; hair of victim and other; saliva; fingernail scrapings; oral, vaginal, and anal swabs and slides (Campbell and Poole 1984)
   f. Assess the patient's mental status:
      - Affect—blunted, depressed, or fearful
      - Defense mechanisms—denial, fear, shame, silence, or anger
      - Memory—recent and remote (the patient may block memories of the incident)
      - Speech patterns
      - Mood—depressed, anxious, or panicked
   g. Identify the patient's resources and sources of emotional support
   h. Assess the patient's immediate concerns
   i. Initiate laboratory tests, including those for sexually transmitted disease, HIV antibody, pregnancy, U/A, CBC, and motile sperm
   j. Conduct a health history
2. Sexual concerns or differences
   a. Conduct a health history—including physical disabilities, medications, and sexual orientation
   b. Identify the patient's concerns
   c. Identify the patient's resources and sources of emotional support. This may include significant others as well as family

B. Planning

Planning as well as treatment should be based on a combination of both a comprehensive nursing assessment and subsequent nursing diagnoses. Modification of the plan should be carried out based on reassessments of the progress of the patient and evaluation of the care given. It is useful to set short- and long-term goals with the patient who has sexual problems.

1. Short-term goals in *crisis intervention* include:
   a. Provide crisis intervention treatment as required initially.
   b. Help the patient cope with loss and grief.
   c. Help the patient understand that there are immediate concerns and that long-term matters can be handled later.
   d. Provide acceptable methods of relieving anxiety and depression.
   e. Help the patient tolerate feelings of loneliness, anger, and helplessness.
   f. Begin a long-term rehabilitation plan as soon as the patient is admitted to the hospital.
2. Long-term goals include helping the patient:
   a. Realize that the goal is a satisfactory sexual and reproductive life for the individual, without forgetting the ability and need to cope with community mores and responsibilities.
   b. Realize that his problems are capable of being dealt with whether on a physical, psychological, social, or other level. Assure the patient, if appropriate, that problems can be handled and that they are not overwhelming.
   c. Discover positive ways to meet personal needs.
   d. Regain self-respect and self-confidence.
   e. Discover positive ways of coping with sexual frustration.
   f. Understand anxiety and depression and when and where to seek help.
   g. Seek new ways of feeling pleasure.

C. Intervention

1. Prevention

By virtue of her role, the nurse can do a great deal by educating patients, students, and people in the community about sexuality, human reproduction, and sexually transmitted diseases. Positive attitudes, enjoyment without violence and infringement on the rights of others, and responsible sex are topics that can be covered.

The nurse should be aware that many people have sexual problems and that such factors as alcoholism, narcotics use, depression, physical pathology, and stress can decrease desire and arousal mechanisms and limit the ability to achieve satisfactory completion of the sexual act. Educational material should be offered to patients who have spinal cord injuries, cardiac disease, multiple sclerosis and other neurological diseases, diabetes, and any other physical conditions that may affect sexual functioning. Overanxiety, religious teachings, psychosomatic disorders, and poor communication with a partner all can contribute to sexual failure. Some educational or preventive interventions by the nurse can eliminate such problems; other problems can better be solved through therapeutic programs.

School and community groups should be informed about sexual abuse, preventive measures, and procedures for reporting incidents.

Teach children to be cautious of strangers and to be very wary of *anyone* who makes sexual advances.

Make children aware of their personal rights and the elements of healthy family relationships.

Publicize telephone numbers for crisis and sexual assault programs.

Commonsense behavior should be emphasized:

a. Avoid dark streets and parking lots.
b. Travel with companions, not alone.
c. Be cautious of strangers who come to the door, especially those seeking entrance.
d. Be careful about information given over the phone to strangers.
e. Walk with head up and be alert to the environment.
f. Parents should give children a "secret code": if a stranger offers a child a ride and does not know the "code," the child should be instructed to refuse the ride.

2. Treatment

Treatment of sexual problems can be graduated from simple reassurances to long-term programs in therapeutic clinics specializing in sexual problems. Many excellent books, articles, reports, and films are available about treatment programs. The nurse should be very aware of these programs and about when to refer patients for help at them. However, the nurse should not expect that only experts can solve problems. There are many treatment interventions that can be carried out by the nurse.

A general plan of action includes a behavioral assessment and a behavioral intervention program. The latter might use psychological and behavioral methods to increase desired sexual responses through providing information, modifying "shoulds" and "musts," changing stimuli that have been associated with failure, encouraging positive reinforcement by changing performance expectations, using systematic desensitization to reduce anxiety, and retraining through modeling, role-playing, and instructions. Such a plan might also train the client to avoid certain situations, be more sensitive to unwanted behavior, and use aversive conditioning to avoid problems (Fischer and Gochros 1977).

3. Medications

   A number of medications may interfere with sexual functioning, including:

   a. Tricyclic antidepressants
   b. Major tranquilizers
   c. Cimetidine
   d. Beta-blockers
   e. Various antihypertensive agents (thiazides, methyldopa)
   f. Anabolic steroids
   g. Lithium

4. Nursing Actions

   a. Patients with alternative lifestyles
      - Be aware of personal beliefs and prevent them from interfering with the nurse-patient relationship
      - Respect the patient's right to choose an alternative lifestyle
      - Maintain confidentiality.
      - Keep the patient safe and protect him from harassment from others with differing beliefs.

   b. Victims (survivors of sexual abuse or trauma crisis)
      - Because many people have negative feelings toward persons with sexual differences, and these feelings can interfere with treatment, it is essential that the nurse be attuned to her personal feelings toward sexuality and persons who may be different in their sexual behaviors.
      - Recovery can proceed best when the patient recognizes and talks about problems. The patient should be encouraged to recognize and talk about concerns. Do not evade the discussion if a patient wishes to talk about his problems. Allow the patient to express feelings of quietness, anger, rage, and shame.
      - The patient may become aggressive, seductive, or hostile. Provide a safe, protective supervised environment for the patient who is acting in ways that endanger or infringe on others.
      - Keep surroundings as peaceful as possible to decrease anxiety and agitation.
      - Keep patients who have undergone sexual trauma protected and safe from harm. During crisis intervention, a person of the same sex may (but not necessarily) be important to provide treatment; use professional judgment.

- Rape victims should have a complete physical assessment, and medical records should be carefully maintained. Accurate and complete accounts should be recorded for possible court use. Counseling and support are extremely important, and should be provided as needed. Followup is generally desirable.
- If the patient is hospitalized, promote sleep and rest with warm showers at night, hot drinks, and drugs prescribed for sedation. Allow the patient to sleep as long as possible.
- Explain the reasons for all tests and procedures to gain the patient's cooperation and reduce the fear of not knowing what is happening.
- Allow the patient to talk about problems, to express feelings of resentment, hopelessness, guilt, and remorse, and to express rationalizations and alibis. Listen respectfully.
- Do not leave the victim alone. Stay with him until a friend, relative, or crisis counselor can be with the victim.

c. Continuing treatment and convalescence

- Understand that sexuality is pervasive throughout life. Enable the patient to understand this.
- Accept the patient as a worthwhile human. Although the person who has been traumatized has increased feelings of shame, guilt, and worthlessness, do not reinforce these feelings. The person needs to regain or to learn self-worth and dignity.
- Plan regular daily routines to provide an adequate balance of rest, work, socialization, and interaction with others. Patients need to learn to reestablish healthful patterns of living.
- Look for symptoms of depression, which are often an aftermath of sexual trauma.
- Encourage the patient to make personal decisions to cope with life's responsibilities. Teach problem-solving skills. Permanent rehabilitation is facilitated by the patient's decisions to take charge of his own life in a responsible fashion.
- Insist that the patient take part in ward tasks or work assignments. Completing small responsibilities facilitates progression to greater ones.
- Be firm, yet helpful and understanding. Rejection or perceived rejection from the staff inhibits treatment.
- Allow the patient to ventilate anger and hostility. The sexually abused person feels guilt, anger, and resentment.

Expression of these feelings helps the patient deal with them.

- Encourage participation in recreational activities. Activity promotes physical health and helps the patient interact with others and helps disseminate feelings of frustration and anger.
- Give emotional support without being overly sympathetic with the patient. Use a firm, kind, calm, matter-of-fact manner with the patient to prevent manipulation and to avoid the person gaining favors or making excuses for his condition.
- Help the patient focus on strengths and talents. Stressing the patient's worth and positive points helps build a healthy self-image.
- Spend time with the convalescing patient to allay loneliness.
- Provide diversions. Too much unstructured time is a hindrance to recovery.
- Refer to agency or community resources for followup care after discharge.
- Encourage the patient to help others with the same problems. Helping others provides strength, reinforcement, and satisfaction to the recovering individual.
- As recovery occurs, make the patient increasingly responsible for himself or herself. Start with appointments, personal hygiene, meals, and so on. The primary treatment is to help the patient meet life's responsibilities. This begins with small responsibilities and progresses to greater responsibilities.

d. Patients demonstrating seductive or sexually acting-out behavior

- Be aware of personal feelings such as anger or discomfort when patients display these behaviors.
- Observe for symptoms of underlying mental illness or personality disorders that can lead to violence, aggression, seduction, and so on.
- When appropriate, confront the patient who is manipulative. The seducer is often a "con artist," skilled at flattering staff to obtain favors and talented at obtaining special privileges or getting staff to overlook infractions of the rules.
- Promote participation in ward activities and recreational activities.
- Prevent the patient from playing one staff member against another by formulating a treatment plan, being consistent, and setting appropriate limits.

- Communicate clear, consistent, and firm expectations for behavior.
- If the patient is acting out in a sexually inappropriate manner, such as masturbating in view of others, explain in a matter-of-fact, nonjudgmental manner that this behavior is inappropriate. Provide diversional activities to structure the patient's time and to decrease his anxiety.
- Do not accept the patient's explanations and reassurances if and when bragging about exploits. Individuals can cleverly camouflage problems and behavior with rationalization and minimization. At times, the patient seems so rational that it is deceivingly tempting to try reason. Be careful to listen not only to what you are hearing, but also to what you are not *hearing*.
- Encourage the patient to tone down superior attitudes, which are often a defense to avoid dealing with real feelings of guilt, shame, and inadequacy. Sometimes a superior attitude is used as an excuse to avoid working in treatment.
- Help the patient focus on his strengths.
- Encourage the patient to assume responsibility for himself and his behavior.

D. Evaluation/Expected Outcomes

Effective nursing management can be evaluated in terms of observable behaviors.

1. The nurse will:
   a. Provide an emotionally warm and stable environment.
   b. Meet physical (physiological) needs of the patient until he can do this.
   c. Gradually increase levels of responsibility to be handled by the patient.
2. The patient will:
   a. Learn, realize, and understand the facts and accept them as being self-applicable.
   b. Learn and practice the constructive use of time.
   c. Take increasing responsibility for activities of daily living.
   d. Interact with staff and other patients, family, and friends.
   e. Identify and evaluate feelings, behavior, and situations that precipitate desirable and undesirable behaviors, and seek to bring about appropriate personal changes.
   f. Identify and verbalize personal strengths. Build a positive self-image.
   g. Become involved in ongoing therapy.

h. Learn techniques for self-protection.
i. Be able to continue or become involved in intimate relationships.

E. Evaluation for Referral

Patients who have special sexual difficulties, who have experienced sexual trauma, or who have been charged with sexual offenses should be referred for follow-up and therapy to community or private psychiatric/psychological facilities that specialize in this type of treatment.

IV. POTENTIAL NURSING DIAGNOSES

1. Anxiety (moderate to panic), related to
   - feelings of helplessness
   - fear
   - concern about physical functioning
   - lack of knowledge
   - feelings of shame or humiliation
   - lack of trust
   - intrusive thoughts
2. Injury, potential for, related to
   - abusive behavior
   - substance abuse
   - anger
   - hostility
   - history of dysfunctional or abusive relationships
3. Rape Trauma Syndrome, related to
   - anger
   - unresolved feelings
   - guilt
   - depression
   - sense of helplessness (see Chapter 5, "The Patient with Post-Traumatic Stress Disorder")
4. Self-concept, disturbance in, related to
   - low self-esteem
   - guilt
   - feelings of inadequacy
5. Sexual dysfunction, related to
   - fear
   - changes in health status
   - situational or personal crisis
   - disordered thought processes

V. SUMMARY

Sexuality is a basic and important influence in the lives of all human beings. Problems involving sexuality can be related to situational or maturational crises, change in health status, unconscious conflict about essential values and goals, differing beliefs, and assault or trauma. Sexuality is often a topic of embarrassment and therefore avoided by many health care professionals. It is, however, an area of major concern to patients and should be considered in providing holistic patient care.

References

Campbell, J., and Poole, N. K. (1984). Person abuse. In J. Howe, E. G. Dickason, D. A. Jones, and M. J. Snider (Eds.), *The handbook of nursing.* New York: John Wiley & Sons.

Clinard, M. B., and Meier, R. F. (1975). *Sociology of deviant behavior.* New York: Holt, Rinehart and Winston.

D'Augelli, A., and D'Augelli, J. F. (1985). The enhancement of sexual skills and competence: Promoting lifelong sexual unfolding. In L. L'Abate and M. Milan (Eds.), *Handbook of social skills training and research.* New York: John Wiley & Sons.

Fischer, J., and Gochros, H. L. (1977). *Handbook of behavior therapy with sexual problems. Volume 1—General procedures.* New York: Pergamon Press.

Haber, J., Schudy, S. M., Leach, A. M., et al. (1978). *Comprehensive psychiatric nursing.* New York: McGraw-Hill.

Honea, S. W., and Durrett, B. H. (1984). Psychiatric emergencies. In J. Howe, E. G. Dickason, D. A. Jones, and M. J. Snider (Eds.), *The handbook of nursing.* New York: John Wiley & Sons.

Institute for Information Studies. (1982). *Intimacy and disability.* Falls Church, VA: The Institute.

Kaplan, H. S. (1979). *Disorders of sexual desire and other new concepts and techniques in sex therapy.* New York: Simon and Schuster.

Kilmann, P. R., and Mills, K. M. (1983). *All about sex therapy.* New York: Plenum Press.

Kim, M. J., McFarland, G., and McLane, A. (Eds.). (1984). *Classification of nursing diagnoses: Proceedings of the fifth national conference.* St. Louis: C. V. Mosby.

Kinsey, A. C., Pomeroy, W. B., and Martin, C. E. (1948). *Sexual behavior in the human male.* Philadelphia: Saunders.

Kinsey, A. C., Pomeroy, W. B., and Gebhard, P. H. (1953). *Sexual behavior in the human female.* Philadelphia: Saunders.

LoPiccolo, J., and LoPiccolo, L. (Eds.). (1978). *Handbook of sex therapy.* New York and London: Plenum Press.

LoPiccolo, J., and Miller, V. H. (1975). A program for enhancing the sexual relationship of normal couples. *The Counseling Psychologist, 5,* 41–45.

Masters, W. H., and Johnson, V. E. (1966). *Human sexual response.* Boston: Little, Brown.

Masters, W. H., and Johnson, V. E. (1970). *Human sexual inadequacy.* Boston: Little, Brown.

Qualls, C. B., Wincze, J. P., and Barlow, D. H. (1978). *The prevention of sexual disorders: Issues and approaches.* New York: Plenum Press.

Sarrel, L. J., and Sarrel, P. M. (1979). *Sexual unfolding: Sexual development and sex therapies in late adolescence.* Boston: Little, Brown.

Chapter 15

The Patient with A Chronic Illness

Roberta L. Messner

I. STATEMENT OF PURPOSE

Chronic illness is America's most prevalent health problem and represents a major focus for nurses, who must maintain the delicate balance between high-tech/high-touch in the delivery of care. Technological advances not only have increased longevity of life and therefore the incidence of chronic illness, but also have threatened the personalization of health care delivery. The caring nursing touch is vital to preserving balance in chronic illness.

The purpose of this chapter is twofold:

- To increase the nurse's knowledge and understanding of the trajectory of chronic illness and its impact on the individual, family, and health care system.
- To provide a nursing framework to facilitate optimal management of the patient with a chronic illness.

II. OVERVIEW OF CHRONIC ILLNESS

A. Description of the Illness

The term chronic illness encompasses all physiological or psychological functioning that is permanent or nonreversible, causes disability, or necessitates rehabilitation or ongoing care. A chronic illness may be in the form of a progressive illness with an uncertain course, a long-term illness whose course is controllable by diet and/or medication, or an illness for which treatment is not available.

Chronic illness differs from acute illness in that it is characterized by exacerbations and remissions, threatening both the length and quality of life. A number of chronic illnesses affect an individual's ability to carry out roles and role relationships, impinging on virtually every aspect of day-to-day living. For many individuals, chronic illness represents a legacy of powerlessness and uncertainty.

The impact of a chronic illness on the individual and his significant others is more than the sum total of the physical aspects of the disorder. Nevertheless, despite the range of human responses to chronic illness, the events that occur are quite predictable. While each chronic illness presents its own unique problems and obstacles, some degree of impaired physiological and psychosocial functioning are generally observed.

B. Incidence

Chronic illness, the number one health problem in the United States (Strauss and Glaser 1975), knows no age boundaries. Approximately 225,000 people or 10% of all individuals in the United States have one or more chronic illnesses, the majority of whom are elderly, but 25% of whom are under 17 years of age (Mitchell 1983). Chronic illness affects males and females equally, both in proportion of the population as well as in degree of limitation (Mitchell 1983).

C. Clinical Manifestations

1. Physiological manifestations of chronic illness are disease-specific and are therefore beyond the scope of this chapter. Strategies for coping with chronic illness, although highly individualized according to traditional coping patterns and the demands of the illness itself, include (Viney and Westbrook 1984):
   a. *Action strategies* (such as information seeking)
   b. *Control strategies* (such as developing mastery over the situation)
   c. *Escape strategies* (such as avoidance or denial)
   d. *Fatalism strategies* (such as resigning one's situation "to the way that life is going to be anyway")
   e. *Optimism strategies* (such as positive thinking)
   f. *Interpersonal coping strategies* (such as talking with friends)
2. As the individual with a chronic illness grieves his loss of health, roles, and role relationships, he experiences many "little deaths" along the way. This process of grieving helps the individual to integrate his losses. The loss and grieving process as classically described by Kübler-Ross for confronting a terminal illness are typical in chronic illness as well. These characteristic behaviors represent a continuum throughout the remissions and exacerbations of chronic illness:

   a. Denial
   b. Anger
   c. Bargaining
   d. Depression
   e. Acceptance
3. The following behaviors may be observed in individuals of all age groups who are coping with a serious, chronic illness and may be intensified during critical developmental stages of the life cycle such as adolescence (Gunther 1984).
   a. *Affect*—anxiety, guilt, surprise, resentment, helplessness, hopelessness, and depression.
   b. *Fear*—fear of separation from loved ones, fear of the unknown and an uncertain future, and fear of discomfort and treatment regimens.
   c. *Regression*—return to less mature behavior.
   d. *Introversion*—withdrawal; self-protective, narcissistic behavior with temporary loss of interest in usual roles, relationships, and activities.
   e. *Attitudes toward medical care-givers*—attitudes are typically a combination of dependency, trust, and hope, alternating with anger, disappointment, and resentment.
   f. *Aggression*—aggressive feelings related to physical restriction, regression, and feelings of helplessness. Aggression may be demonstrated in reaction formation or passive-aggressive behaviors.
   g. *Defensive functioning*—regression, withdrawal, ritualistic behavior, reaction formation, magical thinking, denial, projection, and turning against self.

III. NURSING MANAGEMENT

Comprehensive nursing management of the individual with a chronic illness includes assessment, planning, intervention, and evaluation.

A. Assessment

A comprehensive, ongoing assessment of the individual/family facing chronic illness includes an assessment of the individual's perception of the chronic illness, level of self-esteem, effectiveness of coping strategies, available human and material resources, degree of vulnerability, and potential for crisis.

1. *Perception of the chronic illness*—How an individual/family adapts to the many losses inherent in chronic illness is determined to a large degree by their unique perception of those

losses. For some individuals, the major concern is the effect of the chronic illness on a particular aspect of self. For example, in an illness where body appearance is altered, self-image is affected and the individual may feel unattractive or inadequate. If body function is impaired, this may distort perception, giving a feeling of being incomplete and unable to perform at a former level of functioning. Prosthetic devices may call attention to a handicap.

2. *Level of self-esteem*—Positive self-esteem facilitates participation in health promotion and self-care activities, enhances the potential for successful and confident role performance, and provides the individual with more accurate feedback about self. Individuals with low self-esteem prior to the diagnosis of a chronic illness are thought to be increasingly vulnerable to low self-esteem during the illness. The level of self-esteem can be assessed by noting verbal and nonverbal communication.
3. *Effectiveness of coping strategies*—Coping strategies are the customary ways in which an individual/family adapts to stressful events in an attempt to maintain balance and avoid crisis. Coping mechanisms are based on the individual's past experiences and include denial; selective ignoring; information seeking; taking refuge in activity; avoidance; reminiscence about former good times; learning specific illness-related tasks; blaming others; seeking comfort from others; and the utilization of spiritual resources. The nurse should assess the adequacy of the individual's coping strategies in meeting disease-imposed demands as well as possible suicidal or homicidal ideation.
4. *Available human and material resources*—This includes an appraisal of the individual's financial and "people" resources as well as his cultural and social orientation.
5. *Degree of vulnerability*—Assessment of vulnerability is an important part of the nursing assessment, as the nurse frequently intervenes during periods of increased vulnerability. This is helpful in anticipatory planning and in developing crisis prevention strategies. Individuals who are more vulnerable include those with a history of ineffectual coping and low self-esteem and those lacking vital human and material resources. Periods of increased vulnerability include at the time of diagnosis; as the illness progresses (change in symptoms, impingement on lifestyle, or hospitalization); and during maturational and situational crises.
6. *Potential for crisis*—The nurse should assess visible signs of crisis, such as anxiety, chaotic thinking, depression, or behavioral changes (such as increased conflict), and the resources available to meet the demands of the crisis. The severity of the

crisis, particularly suicidal or homicidal ideation, and deterioration of the patient's condition should be carefully assessed.

B. Planning

Planning of nursing intervention is based on a comprehensive nursing assessment and the development of subsequent nursing diagnoses. Nursing care is based on principles of rehabilitation and not on expectations of cure. This approach focuses on maximizing current resources and helping the individual to procure additional needed resources.

C. Intervention

1. Prevention

   A major thrust of nursing care for the individual facing a chronic illness is the prevention and early recognition of crises and keeping identified crises within manageable limits.

   Potential crises may be averted by the timely assessment of strengths and weaknesses that may influence the coping process and utilization of appropriate nursing strategies (i.e., encouraging expression of feelings, providing information about the illness and its treatment, enhancing communication, and facilitating anticipatory planning).

2. Treatment

   Treatment of the individual with a chronic illness far exceeds the remission or control of disease. It involves addressing the multifaceted needs of the individual and his significant others.

   a. *Crisis Management.* In situations of potential suicide, homicide, or deterioration of the patient's condition, timely, situation-specific intervention assumes paramount importance. The goals of crisis intervention are resolution of the crisis or restoration of functioning to at least the precrisis level, and ideally with some promotion of growth.

   b. *Pain and Symptom Management.* Pain and symptom management are disease-specific for each chronic illness. The nurse should understand that there is a psychological dimension to pain and other symptoms and that the individual's past experiences with symptoms may exert a profound influence on his current symptoms. Timely and judicious use of analgesics and other medicinal agents coupled with reassurance are important. A sensitive, individualized nursing approach is crucial. Nonmedical interventions such as mental imagery, progressive relaxation, and the use of distraction (giving the individual something else to occupy his thoughts) are often beneficial in the management of chronic pain and other symptoms (see also Chapter 20, "Psychotropic Medications").

3. Medications

   Medications prescribed for various chronic illnesses are generally disease-specific and will not be discussed in great detail. Assessment of chronic pain and other symptoms is often both challenging and difficult. Medications, however, represent only one approach to the management of chronic pain. Effective nurse/patient communication is essential to enhance understanding of the patient's symptoms. Antidepressants may be given as adjuncts to pain medications, since when an individual is depressed, his perception of pain may be heightened. Antidepressants may also raise the pain threshold in some individuals.

4. Nursing Actions

   It is beyond the scope of this chapter to list all nursing interventions for the patient/family experiencing chronic illness. Each individual is unique and therefore possesses a unique set of clinical manifestations and a unique psychosocial constellation. The promotion of optimal health, based on the nursing process, is the goal toward which the efforts of nursing are directed. Generalized nursing interventions are as follows:

   a. Establish rapport with patient/family as early as possible. This is facilitated by setting aside time to listen and communicating genuine interest and caring.
   b. Assess the patient/family's perception of the chronic illness, level of self-esteem, customary coping mechanisms, and available support systems.
   c. Help the patient/family to recognize and utilize available internal and external resources and assist the patient to discover and mobilize new resources.
   d. Help the patient/family to become more aware of and eliminate negative self-talk.
   e. Identify periods of increased vulnerability and impending crisis and provide appropriate anticipatory guidance in regard to potential maturational and situational crises.
   f. Help the patient/family to grieve and work through the losses of chronic illness and disability (health, independence, certainty, control, self-esteem, usual roles and role relationships, productivity, financial security, sexuality, and appearance).
   g. Help the patient/family to learn to live with the uncertainties of chronic illness and integrate the management and changing demands of chronic illness into their family life-

style, perceiving the patient *not* as disabled but as differently-abled. This is facilitated by the establishment of short-term and long-term goals.

h. Assist the patient/family to identify and utilize effective coping strategies to enhance adaptation to chronic illness, accepting what cannot be changed, maximizing positive experiences of daily living (turning obstacles into opportunities), and finding strength in weaknesses.
i. Teach the patient/family alternative, nonmedicinal measures for pain and symptom control (i.e., relaxation techniques, mental imagery, positive thinking, and humor).
j. To increase the patient's capability for self-care, provide appropriate patient/family education in regard to the course and management of the chronic illness and to the signs and symptoms that warrant seeking medical intervention.
k. Educate the patient/family regarding gaining access to and utilization of the health care system.
l. Initiate appropriate referrals to community resources and supportive networks.
m. Offer psychological support, reassurance, understanding, and unconditional professional caring.
n. Foster the patient's independence and maintenance of usual roles and role relationships as much as possible within the context of the chronic "sick role."
o. Employ strategies to enhance self-esteem and diminish social isolation.
p. Help the patient/family maintain hope and a sense of control in the midst of uncertainty.

D. Evaluation/Expected Outcomes

Effective nursing management will be evaluated in terms of the patient/family's adaptation to the chronic illness.

1. The nurse will:
   a. Monitor physiological and psychosocial adaptation to chronic illness, providing task-oriented assistance and anticipatory guidance.
   b. Minimize patient/family vulnerability by maximizing internal and external resources.
   c. Identify behavior indicating actual or potential crises.
2. The patient/family will:
   a. Demonstrate an adequate knowledge base regarding the nature and course of the illness and the signs and symptoms that warrant seeking medical intervention.

b. Operationalize coping strategies that are flexible and reality-oriented, facilitate the expression of feelings, and are effective in managing chronic illness.

E. Evaluation for Referral

The patient/family should be assessed in regard to their perception of the chronic illness and its effect on life and self as well as their available time and material resources. "People" resources for possible referral include clergy, social workers, nurse practitioners, and self-help or support groups.

IV. POTENTIAL NURSING DIAGNOSES

Because the term chronic illness encompasses virtually any recurrent health problem characterized by exacerbations and remissions, potential nursing diagnoses are voluminous. This list of actual or potential nursing diagnoses is limited to those psychosocial diagnoses and physical diagnoses with a psychosocial component most commonly encountered (Kim et al. 1984).

1. Activity intolerance/Diversional activity deficit, related to
   - physical debilitation
   - depression
   - disinterest
2. Anxiety (mild, moderate, severe) related to
   - feelings of fear
   - hopelessness
   - helplessness
   - impaired thought processes associated with illness
3. Body image disturbance, related to
   - physical changes associated with illness
   - depression
4. Bowel elimination, alteration in, related to
   - physiological effects of illness
   - anxiety
5. Conflict, decisional; unresolved independence-dependence, related to
   - imposed dependence on health care givers
   - feelings of helplessness

6. Cognitive impairment, related to
   - anxiety
   - depression
   - decreased mental activity
   - physiological changes
7. Comfort, alteration in, related to
   - pain
   - physiological changes
   - medication side effects
   - altered sleep patterns
8. Communication, impaired verbal, related to
   - physiological changes
   - depression
   - loss of memory and language skills
9. Consciousness, altered levels of, related to
   - medications
   - effects of illness
10. Contractures, related to immobility: self-imposed associated with depression or illness-related restrictions on movement
11. Coping, ineffectual individual/family, related to
    - anxiety
    - altered thought processes
    - feelings of helplessness
    - role changes
12. Gas exchange, impaired, related to pulmonary disease
13. Grieving, dysfunctional: anticipatory, related to
    - feelings of hopelessness
    - impotence
    - helplessness
    - losses
14. Home maintenance management, impaired: alienation related to dependency effects on interpersonal relationships
15. Infection, potential for, related to
    - generalized physical debilitation
    - deficient immune system
16. Injury, potential for, related to
    - physical weakness
    - musculoskeletal or neurologic impairment
    - depression
    - thoughts of suicide
    - apathy
    - impaired thought processes associated with illness and/or medication effects

17. Knowledge deficit, related to
    - denial
    - impaired thought processes
18. Mobility, impaired physical, related to illness-associated restrictions
19. Noncompliance, related to
    - depression
    - denial
    - altered thought processes
    - lack of physical means
20. Nutrition, alteration in, related to
    - anorexia associated with illness
    - medication side effects or depression
    - increased or decreased requirements associated with illness
21. Pain related to physical changes
22. Parenting, alteration in, related to
    - preoccupation with self and needs associated with illness
    - depression
    - anxiety
    - physiological changes
23. Powerlessness, related to imposed dependency on health care givers
24. Self-care deficit, related to
    - physical debilitation
    - depression
    - disinterest
25. Self-concept, disturbance in, related to
    - physiological changes (real or imagined)
    - depression
    - feelings of worthlessness
26. Sensory deficit, related to
    - illness
    - impaired mental acuity
27. Sexuality patterns, altered, related to
    - physiological changes
    - depression
    - anxiety
28. Skin integrity, impaired, related to
    - nutrition deficit
    - immobility

29. Sleep pattern disturbance, related to
    - pain
    - medication
    - anxiety
    - depression
30. Social isolation, related to
    - restrictions imposed by illness
    - feelings of worthlessness
    - fear of others' reactions to illness
31. Spiritual distress, related to
    - fear of dying
    - fear of pain
    - feelings of despair
    - depression
32. Thought processes, alteration in, related to
    - depression
    - anxiety
    - effects of illness or medications
33. Urinary elimination, alteration in patterns of, related to genitourinary impairment
34. Violence, potential for, related to
    - impaired thought processes
    - anger
    - depression

V. SUMMARY

The concepts and strategies presented in this chapter provide the nurse with a holistic framework for intervention in chronic illness. For the individual with a chronic illness, the nursing focus is on care rather than cure. This involves helping the patient not only to cope with the illness and its accompanying symptoms, but also to cope with life as it is altered by chronic illness. As such, chronic illness exemplifies the tremendous human potential for growth even in the midst of uncertainty and adversity.

References

Gunther, M. S. (1984). Acute-onset serious chronic organic illness in adolescence: Some critical issues. *Adolescent Psychiatry, 12,* 59–76.

Kim, M. J., McFarland, G. K., and McLane, A. M. (1984). *Pocket guide to nursing diagnoses.* St. Louis: C. V. Mosby Co.

Leavitt, M. B. (1982). *Families at risk: Family prevention in nursing practice.* Boston: Little, Brown and Company.

Meshil, M. H. (1981). The measurement of uncertainty in illness. *Nursing Research, 30*(5), 258–263.

Mitchell, P. H. (1983). Crisis management for families living with chronic illness. *Washington State Journal of Nursing, 54*(2), 2–8.

Strauss, A. L., and Glaser, B. G. (1975). *Chronic illness and the quality of life.* St. Louis: C. V. Mosby Co.

Viney, L. L., and Westbrook, M. T. (1984). Coping with chronic illness: Strategy preferences, changes in preference and associated emotional reactions. *Journal of Chronic Diseases, 37*(6), 489–502.

Chapter 16

The Patient with AIDS/HIV Infection

Theodore B. Feldmann

I. STATEMENT OF PURPOSE

Acquired immune deficiency syndrome (AIDS) is an illness that represents a major public health problem. In fact, the Surgeon General of the U.S. Public Health Service calls AIDS the greatest health threat of this century. It is a disease of viral etiology for which no effective treatment currently exists. The outcome of the illness is almost always fatal. As a result, AIDS has been the focus of intense media attention. While this attention often serves to educate the public about the risk of AIDS, it has also generated tremendous fear and anxiety affecting not only the general public but also all health care providers. Since the appearance of this disease in 1981, a tremendous amount has been learned about it. In spite of that knowledge, misconceptions and irrational fears abound. These feelings often unduly influence the attitudes and reactions of care-givers toward AIDS patients.

This chapter is designed to present an overview of AIDS and human immunodeficiency virus (HIV) infection from a neuropsychiatric/psychosocial frame of reference to assist the nurse in dealing with these patients. Several key areas will be addressed: (1) the etiology and epidemiology of AIDS, (2) physical and neuropsychiatric manifestations of the disorder, and (3) psychosocial issues facing AIDS patients and their families, friends, and health care providers.

II. OVERVIEW OF AIDS

A. Description of the Illness

AIDS is an infection transmitted via the exchange of blood or body fluids. It attacks an individual's immune system, rendering him incapable of fighting off various infections to which a healthy individual is generally resistant. It also interferes with the immune system's ability to defend against the development of certain types of cancer. Thus the person infected with AIDS is at increased risk to develop opportunistic infections (e.g., *Pneumocystis carinii* pneumonia) or malignancies (e.g., Kaposi's sarcoma). It is the body's inability to fight off these other illnesses that results in the extremely high mortality rate of AIDS.

The illness has now been found to be caused by a viral agent referred to as the human immunodeficiency virus (HIV). This virus enters the blood stream and attacks certain of the white blood cells, specifically the T lymphocytes, which play a key role in the immune system. By damaging these lymphocytes, the AIDS virus seriously compromises the immune system. In response to infection with the AIDS virus, the body produces antibodies, which are used in a screening test to determine whether or not an individual is infected. Antibody seroconversion generally takes from 6–12 weeks. Complicating this scenario is the fact that the AIDS virus has a long incubation period, ranging from 8 months to 4 years or longer.

In addition to the various clinical manifestations of AIDS, a number of intense psychosocial stresses accompany the illness. Much of the psychosocial impact of AIDS is influenced by the intense fear generated by the disease. Nearly every aspect of the patient's life is affected by the disease. The coping skills of the patient are severely tested by these stresses.

In some respects, AIDS creates psychosocial problems similar to those encountered by terminal cancer patients. Clearly the presence of a life-threatening illness provides a major stress. Intensifying this stress, however, is the fact that no effective treatment exists for the underlying immunodeficiency. A variety of other factors also make the impact of AIDS greater than is the case with other life-threatening illnesses. First, AIDS predominantly attacks individuals with certain lifestyle charcteristics, namely, those with homosexual or bisexual lifestyles and intravenous drug users. In many segments of the population, considerable stigma exists around these lifestyles. AIDS also may appear relatively quickly, with rapid progression and deterioration in previously healthy persons. Most AIDS patients are between 25 and 49 years of age, an age group that does not usually develop fatal illnesses. These factors, and many others, make the psychosocial impact of AIDS unique.

B. Incidence

The first case of AIDS was described in 1981. Since then the disease has reached epidemic proportions. According to statistics released by the Centers for Disease Control (CDC), as of Feb. 20, 1989, over 87,188 cases of AIDS had been reported. Of these cases there were 49,976 deaths. The Surgeon General projects that by the end of 1991 there will be 270,000 cases diagnosed, with a cumulative total of 365,000 cases by the end of 1992. Many investigators, however, feel that these projections may be low. Adding to the magnitude of the problem is the fact that between one and two million Americans are thought to be infected with HIV (i.e., are seropositive), an unknown number of whom will eventually develop the disease.

C. Clinical Manifestations

AIDS has now been recognized to be the final stage of a spectrum of illness. This sequence proceeds from infection with the causative agent (antibody seroconversion) to development of the AIDS-related complex (ARC), with final progression to the development of AIDS itself, although an individual does not necessarily progress through each of these stages. ARC is a variant of AIDS infection in which the patient tests positive for exposure to AIDS and has specific clinical symptoms, but these are less severe than the life-threatening infections and malignancies associated with AIDS. It is unclear how many patients with ARC will go on to develop AIDS.

As more is learned about AIDS and its clinical manifestations, the importance of neuropsychiatric manifestations in the presentation of the illness is being appreciated. Recent research has shown that the AIDS virus can directly infect the central nervous system, leading to a variety of neuropsychiatric symptoms.

1. Physical signs and symptoms of ARC include, but are not limited to: Decreased appetite, fever, weight loss, night sweats, skin rashes, fatigue, lack of resistance to infection, and enlarged lymph nodes.
2. Neurological manifestations of AIDS include: headache; encephalopathy; meningitis; weakness and paresthesias; seizures; ataxia; incontinence; peripheral neuropathies; and a variety of focal neurological signs.
3. Specific psychological/psychosocial manifestations of AIDS include the following:
   a. Delirium and dementia are common findings in AIDS patients. Several cases have been reported in which dementia was the initial symptom, appearing long before AIDS was suspected.
   b. Depression is common in AIDS patients. This may represent a psychological reaction to having a life-threatening

illness, or it may represent an organic affective disorder secondary to infection of the brain.

c. Mania is also seen in AIDS patients, again representing an organic affective disorder.
d. Personality changes are frequently seen in AIDS patients. This may often be the first symptom observed and may be noticed before AIDS is suspected.
e. Adjustment disorders with either anxious or depressed mood are by far the most frequent psychiatric diagnoses seen in AIDS patients. The tremendous psychological impact of this illness makes the development of an adjustment disorder easily understandable.
f. A diagnosis of AIDS or ARC in itself presents a major psychosocial stress. The patient must face the reality of having an illness that is usually fatal. Those patients with ARC face uncertainty about whether or not they will develop AIDS. Likewise, individuals who are seropositive also experience tremendous anxiety related to their chances of developing this disease. There have been a number of case reports of suicide among patients recently diagnosed with AIDS or ARC, and those found to be seropositive.
g. Many lifestyle changes are associated with AIDS. The patient must begin to deal with the fact that his life will no longer be the same. Frequent hospitalizations will likely be necessary, accompanied by often painful treatments and procedures. Limitations in physical activity must be dealt with, as well as the need to take exceptional precautions against acquiring an opportunistic infection.
h. AIDS has a significant effect on employment and insurance coverage. Patients are often physically unable to work because of the illness. In other instances, patients may be fired from their jobs because of irrational fears on the part of their employers. All of this may lead to loss of health insurance coverage at a time when it is needed most. This only adds to the fears and concerns that these patients must face. Serious financial problems often arise for the patient and the family.
i. Considerable guilt is experienced by AIDS patients. This often involves unresolved feelings over lifestyle as well as regret over things not accomplished in life.
j. Relationships are often profoundly affected. Concern about infecting sexual partners is frequent. Abandonment by family and friends is also a common fear.
k. Identity and self-image are greatly affected by the illness. Some patients tend to view themselves as flawed or imper-

fect. Others react with feelings of inadequacy. The loss of physical abilities or mental faculties further intensifies this alteration of self-image.

l. Fear of AIDS in the general public and/or disapproval of certain lifestyles often leads to discrimination against AIDS patients. Even health care providers often react in a negative or hostile manner to AIDS patients. These reactions create intense pressures on the patient.

m. Family conflicts are commonly seen in association with this illness. In many instances the family has been unaware of the patient's lifestyle. In addition to dealing with a critical illness, the family must also deal with feelings about the lifestyle. This family conflict unfortunately occurs at a time when the patient needs the support of family and friends the most.

III. NURSING MANAGEMENT

A. Assessment

Assessment of the patient with HIV infection is based on the aforementioned clinical manifestations. Assessment of the individual at risk for HIV infection is based on the individual's participation in high-risk behaviors. There are three modes of transmission for the virus: (1) sexual (particularly those who have engaged in anal-receptive intercourse), (2) parenteral, and (3) perinatal. The main risk groups are homosexuals (males are at greater risk than homosexual females), intravenous (IV) drug users, heterosexual females who have male partners infected with the virus, and children born to infected mothers. In the past, individuals receiving blood transfusions were at high risk, but now procedures to safely screen blood for the virus have been developed, thus minimizing that risk. It is important to remember that AIDS is not transmitted by casual contact, through the air, or by household pets. Only direct contact involving the exchange of body fluids poses a significant risk.

B. Planning

Planning of care for the patient with AIDS is highly individualized and based on the clinical manifestations/phase of the illness and information obtained from the nursing assessment.

C. Intervention

1. Prevention

The most effective measure of preventing AIDS is education. All individuals should become aware of the dangers posed by this illness. Since AIDS is often transmitted through sexual contact, safe sexual practices should be taught to all those participating in high-risk behaviors. Because heterosexuals are increasingly at risk for AIDS, education should not be limited to the homosexual community. The dangers of needle-sharing by IV drug users should likewise be emphasized.

To prevent transmission of the AIDS virus in the health care setting, health care professionals should institute universal isolation precautions (e.g., hand washing, wearing of gloves, and other appropriate barrier precautions) when handling the blood and body fluids of *all* patients, being mindful that AIDS is not transmitted through the air or by casual contact. The excessive use of masks or gowns is unnecessary and serves only to stigmatize patients.

Note: While AIDS is not transmitted by casual contact, AIDS hysteria can be.

Hospital infection control procedures should be based on the premise that the blood and body fluids of *all* patients are potentially infectious, not just those of patients known to have a bloodborne infectious disease. Therefore, gloves should be worn whenever exposure to blood or body fluids of *any* patient is anticipated. Gowns should be worn when splashing of blood or body fluids is anticipated. Similarly, masks/goggles should be worn if aerosolization of blood or body fluids is anticipated. Hands should be washed after any patient or body substance contact, even if gloves have been worn. These precautions warrant special attention in emergency settings, where the risk of blood exposure is increased and the infection status of the patient may not be known (Centers for Disease Control 1987).

2–3. Treatment/Medications

A discussion of the treatment/medications for this disease is beyond the scope of this chapter, but is based on the phase of illness and clinical manifestations. Treatment is aimed at primary health maintenance, secondary health care, or tertiary health care, depending upon the presenting health problems. The reader is referred to the many excellent publications on the subject.

4. Nursing Actions

a. Just as appropriate medical and nursing care is needed to address the physical manifestations of AIDS, attention must be paid to the many psychosocial issues related to the illness. AIDS patients are vulnerable to a variety of physical and psychological complications. By addressing the psychosocial aspects of AIDS, the nurse not only provides better patient care, but also improves the quality of life for these patients and improves the therapeutic relationship with them. For specific nursing actions, please refer to the chapters in this book that deal with pertinent psychosocial issues (e.g., anxiety, depression, and so on).

b. In addition to the psychosocial stresses experienced by AIDS patients and their families and friends, the illness also imposes severe stresses on health care providers that often serve as impediments to rational infection-control practices. These include:
   - Feelings of frustration and helplessness due to the lack of effective treatment and the poor prognosis of the illness.
   - Staff burnout secondary to the intense needs of these patients and the demands created by the severity of the illness.
   - Staff fears about contracting the illness.
   - Negative reactions to the inevitable regression seen in patients with life-threatening illnesses.
   - Grief over the death of AIDS patients after the expenditure of tremendous energy in their treatment.
   - Negative feelings, of either conscious or unconscious origin, about the lifestyles of AIDS victims.

   Please refer to the following chapters for additional nursing actions: Chapter 15, "The Patient with a Chronic Illness," and Chapter 17, "The Patient Who is Dying."

D. Evaluation/Expected Outcomes

Please refer to Chapter 15, "The Patient with a Chronic Illness," and Chapter 17, "The Patient Who is Dying."

E. Evaluation for Referral

Please refer to Chapter 15, "The Patient with a Chronic Illness," and Chapter 17, "The Patient Who is Dying."

IV. POTENTIAL NURSING DIAGNOSES

The reader is referred to the psychosocial-oriented material in Chapter 15, "The Patient with Chronic Illness," and Chapter 17, "The Patient Who is Dying."

V. SUMMARY

AIDS is a new illness with many clinical manifestations that presents unique challenges for all health care providers. The illness has no effective treatment and is almost always fatal. It may present with a variety of physical and neuropsychiatric symptoms. It is also accompanied by a variety of psychosocial issues affecting patients, family members, friends, and care-givers. This illness has reached epidemic proportions and is often surrounded by irrational fears and biases. A full understanding of the illness and its impact is essential for all nurses so that adequate and sensitive care can be provided.

References

Centers for Disease Control (1981–1987). Report on AIDS. *Morbidity and Mortality Weekly Report* (June 1981 through September 1987).

Centers for Disease Control (1987). Recommendations for prevention of HIV transmission in health-care settings. *Morbidity and Mortality Weekly Report* (August 21).

Centers for Disease Control (Feb. 20, 1989). Personal communication.

Christ, G. H., Wiener, L. S., and Moynihan, R. T. (1986). Psychosocial issues in AIDS. *Psychiatric Annals, 16*(3), 173–179.

Cohen, M. A., and Weisman, H. W. (1986). A biopsychosocial approach to AIDS. *Psychosomatics, 27*(2), 245–249.

Perry, S., and Jacobson, P. (1986). Neuropsychiatric manifestations of AIDS-spectrum disorders. *Hospital and Community Psychiatry, 37*(2), 135–142.

Surgeon General's Report on Acquired Immune Deficiency Syndrome (1986). *JAMA, 256*(2), 2784–2789.

Chapter 17

The Patient Who Is Dying

Priscilla F. Leavitt *Susan J. Lewis*
William A. McDowell

I. STATEMENT OF PURPOSE

The emphasis in this chapter is on understanding the needs of the terminally ill patient, particularly as they are evidenced in a general hospital setting. The in-depth treatment of nursing interventions focuses on the role of the nurse as a care-giver.

II. OVERVIEW OF TERMINAL ILLNESS AND CARE

A. Description of the Illness

A patient who has been diagnosed as having a fatal illness may go through three stages of experiencing the facts and fears of his life coming to an end: acute, chronic, and terminal. It is important for the nurse to assess which stage the patient is going through and what tasks are necessary for the patient to complete at each stage.

The first or acute stage is when the diagnosis of a serious illness is suspected or given. Many patients exhibit a great deal of anxiety and agitation, although some withdraw to become silent and morose. Questions and fears are stated or unstated. Treatment and lifestyle changes are suggested.

The second or chronic stage often accompanies remission or comes after the initial shock has turned into a kind of acknowledgment. Often there is a mixture of acceptance and denial as the patient can talk about the illness or even prepare for the future and then shortly seem to go about business as usual, living very much in the present. He is often undergoing treatment and sees himself as sick. He may experience a great deal of hope, even for cure. In this stage the patient's subconscious is integrating the facts of the illness with the identity of the patient. "I am me; alive, playing many roles AND I am sick and I will die and my roles will be ended."

This second stage can be a preparation for the third phase, the terminal phase. A patient is said to be terminal when the physician comes to the end of the treatment(s) and admits there is nothing more he can do. This stage can be the last few months of life or only a few days. Fears, unfinished tasks, saying good-bye, and coming to terms with the fact that death is near become uppermost in the patient's mind. With support this can be a quieting time. Without support it can be a very anxious experience, with fears and agitation increasing.

B. Incidence

Death is universal. Mortality rates vary for different populations; however, those who are elderly or terminally ill are at greater risk than younger, healthier individuals.

C. Clinical Manifestations

Awareness that death is approaching comes from the patient's physical condition and symptoms, results of diagnostic procedures, and references to time limits made by staff. The patient may be aware that he is dying and may want to discuss it, or he may suspect he is dying and attempt to test the nurse's knowledge. Patients may experience a variety of reactions including depression, withdrawal, self-pity, fear, agitation, restlessness, sleep disturbances, or increased demands. Others may appear calm and serene, introspective, and at peace with themselves. Patients tend to waver back and forth through a continuum of emotions during the process of dying, particularly if the illness is chronic rather than acute. A patient who appears to have reached a calm acceptance one day may be angry and demanding or even deny his condition the next.

The presence of the same care-givers with whom the patient and family can identify provides security and continuity.

Both the dying patient and his family seek identification and partnership with someone in order to feel less alone and to decrease the fear of death. Often the nurse is the one sought out for this role because of her close relationship with the patient and family. The nurse provides an opportunity for those who are hurting to express their anger, pain, and fear to someone who will accept them and not be devastated by the expressed feelings. Through sharing these intense experiences with the patient and family at such a critical time in their lives, the nurse may become similar to an extended family member for a time.

The patient's fear of death and loss of control may be evidenced by agitation, restlessness, sleep disturbances, and frequent "calls" at night. Providing comfort and support rather than isolation can reassure the patient.

A dying patient will remain consistent with his basic personality traits. He will approach death in a manner compatible with his approach to life. Sometimes death is welcomed and accepted; sometimes it is denied, feared, or faced with anger and resentment.

In addition to reviewing his life, the dying patient has three tasks: coping with physical symptoms, anticipating the transition to an unknown state, and dealing with impending separation from loved ones and friends. Sharing feelings of fear serves to dilute them, and the unknown becomes less threatening.

When a patient is not told what the future holds, the staff must try to pretend as if he will recover, forcing them to convey a deceiving message. This robs the patient of his right to know about his condition and does not allow him time to prepare for death.

III. NURSING MANAGEMENT

A. Assessment

In order to assess which stage the patient is in and to ascertain the needs, tasks, and coping defenses or resources that any individual patient has, the following assessment questions may be asked.

1. What are the medical diagnoses?
2. When were they given? (How many times? How recently?)
3. By whom were they given? (Dealing with the certainty of death is easier when the diagnosis is heard from a physician.)
4. To whom was the information given (family, patient, or overheard or surmised by the patient)?
5. What does the patient understand about the illness?
6. What does the family understand about the illness?
7. What coping defenses and behaviors is the patient using?
8. Does the patient see physical changes and/or symptoms as resulting from the illness?
9. With whom has the patient discussed the seriousness of the illness?
10. Is the patient still actively involved in his medical treatment or is he going through the motions, exhibiting no hope of benefit or recovery?
11. What level of agitation is present?

12. What fears exist?
13. How much pain is experienced? (Acute pain is obvious, through postural changes, facial grimaces, and so on. Chronic pain can be seen by withdrawal, apathy, depression, irritability, or lack of facial expression.)
14. What information has been received? What is still needed?
15. What preparations for dying (e.g., wills, bequeaths, funeral arrangements, transfer of properties and responsibilities) has the patient made?
16. What role does the patient's spiritual faith or creed play as life is examined or death contemplated?
17. Who can the patient lean on spiritually?
18. Who are the medical and spiritual professionals, caretakers or family members with whom the patient has a special relationship? After whose visit does he seem comforted? Who does he confide in and question?
19. How much control does the patient perceive he has over how he lives the remaining days?
20. Is the patient limiting or wishing to limit contact to one or two close family members? (This may indicate the last days or hours.)
21. Are there any family members who seem unable to give up the dying patient and whose permission to die the patient seems to need?
22. What are the tasks that the patient still needs to do?
23. What hopes does he still have?
24. Does the patient place many requests on care-givers, in order to gain attention? (This may signal a need for someone to sit down and talk with the patient.)
25. What is the patient's ethnic/cultural view of death?
26. What does the patient value?
27. What does the family know about the illness? About the dying process? About the treatment?
28. What does the patient say has reduced pain and stress in the past?
29. How has the patient coped with severe loss or stress in the past?
30. What is the patient's attitude toward pain?

B. Planning

Nursing care for the terminally ill should be based on the nature of the illness and a team assessment of how gradually or suddenly death is likely to come. Since patients often behave in ways that are different than anticipated, frequently scheduled reassessments of patient status and needs should be held. The patient's knowledge of the diagnosis and the style with which he accepts the diagnosis will have considerable effect on the progression of the illness and/or the dying process.

The question of how the hospital, nursing home, or hospice will best fit in with the patient's needs, the family's needs, and the needs for nursing care must all be considered. Often there is a shifting back and forth between settings, and consideration must be given to communicate treatment, progress, and patient and family response to make the care the most helpful.

C. Invervention

1. Prevention

   Because death is inevitable, preventive measures lie in the area of health promotion. Efforts to prevent illness and to maintain or restore health can help to prolong life. Living each day to the fullest and focusing on the quality of life may diminish the fear of death and facilitate its acceptance.

2. Treatment

   Nurses' own expectations and desires about death and dying influence their actions and personal responses to dying patients. All too often they believe that if the "right" things are done, a beautiful, serene, accepted, "right" death can be accomplished. This leads to a determination on the part of caring professionals to get patients to reveal their innermost feelings and fears about death, whether or not they want or need to, and to change these feelings to calm acceptance. Nurses need to exercise caution and allow patients to deal with feelings and issues as they are psychologically ready. Patients often need their defenses. Because nurses care, they want to take away the pain and to make things better, in the process often trying to fix what cannot be fixed.

   Terminal care involves doing much to alleviate suffering and bring comfort, but often it is not enough. It is then that the only help the nurse can offer to those who are in pain is her presence. Often this lack of anything to do that will be helpful causes nursing staff and family members to avoid or abandon the patient. Thus the patient may experience social death long before he physically dies. Good terminal care means avoiding withdrawal from the patient and providing "safe conduct" from life to death.

   Most patients will not reach acceptance, but many will realize that the inevitable time has come. While they may not go in peace, they may be at peace in not denying that death will occur.

Individuals will have their own styles of dying. Some will not "go gentle into that good night" but will want to rage at the injustice of death. Others will want to fight against the realization by living in utter disregard for their illness and its limitations. They choose to die more quickly, but with their "boots on."

Another style is more passive and accepting. Complaints are never heard. These patients, too, are likely to succumb to death sooner, doing what they are expected to.

People who adopt a style that involves humor, questioning, anger at their treatment and physicians, and crying with support from caring others are often noted to live longer.

Each person usually adopts a style of dying like his style of living. It is important that care-givers recognize the particular style and help the patient work within his own framework, utilizing the resources he has.

3. Medications

   For the terminally ill patient who is experiencing pain, medication should be given to provide comfort. In these instances the staff should not worry about addiction, but should hold the patient's comfort and quality of life as a primary goal. Solutions such as liquid morphine or Bromptons cocktail are used with patients in great pain. Intravenous morphine drips may be used. Drugs like Phenergan (promethazine), which potentiate the effects of the narcotics, may be added. With selected patients, antidepressant therapy may be beneficial.

4. Nursing Actions

   After assessing (1) how imminent death is, (2) the patient's and the family's knowledge and coping skills, and (3) the tasks that need yet to be accomplished by the patient, family members, and the nursing or caretaking staff, intervention can be chosen to fit the particular needs the patient or family might have.

   The following section identifies general areas of need felt by the patient and suggests a variety of interventions that could be implemented.

   a. Physial comfort
      - Medication to control the pain. Many practitioners are overly fearful of prescribing a pain medication in adequate doses for fear of addiction. The goal is to give medication before the pain increases. Pain medication should be given at regular intervals rather then PRN to prevent pain from reaching intolerable levels.
      - Frequently check on patients who are too ill to ask for a drink of water, reduction of light or noise, position

changes, or any other uncomfortable condition to be altered.

- Look for special dietary "treats," soft clothing, or comforting objects.

b. Emotional comfort

- Available presence of nursing staff.
- Atmosphere of calmness and control.
- Caring touch.

c. Competence from care-givers

- Explanation from attending physicians about illness (condition) and its likely progression.
- Full explanation of procedures, tests, moves to different wards, or changes in routine by nurses.
- Keep physical touch and voice calm and confident.
- Enhance patient and family confidence in decisions and procedures made by the attending physician. Seek resolution when patient/family members and the physician disagree as to treatment or procedures. Encourage direct communications of patient/family with the attending physician.

d. Control

- Allow the patient to make as many decisions as possible (e.g., when pain medication is needed, the number and timing of visitors, and environmental choices such as temperature, TV, light, or bed position).
- When appropriate, talk with the patient and the family (separately at first) about their wishes for organ transplants, eye enucleation, and extraordinary means of life support, should that decision need to be made.
- Respect the patient's wish to know. Expect such desires to fluctuate. Sometimes many questions are asked at the initial diagnosis. Often there is a period of denial or withdrawal when the patient does not wish to talk about his illness or approaching death. Follow the patient's lead.
- When control of bodily function is lost, ask the patient to do something that he can still control (e.g., change the position of the bed, eat, go to the bathroom, or talk to another patient).
- Often, as death is near, the patient will want to deal with only one or two family members or friends. Help him control his visitors. Posting a "No Visitors" sign may help him achieve this without risking displeasure from family members.

- If the patient has regressed and exhibits increased involvement with himself (hypochrondrias), excluding the reality of what is happening in the external world, anger and/or withdrawal may result. An angry patient may contribute to the isolation he already experiences by behaving unpleasantly so that staff tends to avoid him. This isolation only increases the anxiety about death and the aloneness that the patient feels and is trying to defend against. Structure a stable, predictable environment with limits set so that the patient does not sense that his nurses are frustrated. With predictable limits and consequences, the patient can retain control of his own behavior.
- Help the patient maintain dignity. Being sensitive to the patient's privacy needs, showing consideration for his embarrassment in "undignified" nursing care procedures, and giving him all the help he needs—but not more—will help to convey respect for the patient as a person.

e. Communication

- Avoid the institutional "we." The patient is taking the bath, not the nurse.
- Encourage dialogue between the patient and physician. It can be helpful and efficient for the patient to write down questions as he thinks of them. Sometimes he will write questions that he cannot voice, such as "How long do I have?"
- Find out what is important to the patient (the values with which he has lived) and the special relationships he has. Help him to convey that meaning by suggesting he find a way to let his spouse, a special grandchild, or church/organization know how he feels. Occasionally the nurse may need to "set it up" by suggesting that the patient has something to say to a spouse, for instance, and clearing the room for that stated purpose.

  Listening and suggesting other ways to communicate values can include bequeaths, special information passed on, or telling or writing to a child or grandchild about a guiding principle for his life.
- Be available to listen. The patient's questions about his illness, procedures, and philosophy of life may all be tests to see whether the nurse will talk straight about important topics.
- Honesty is important. It may be particularly difficult at the stage where the patient and/or certain family members have not been told of a terminal diagnosis. Evasive

answers or avoidance, however, only serve to heighten anxiety and communicate that this nurse is not able to be trusted.

- When the subject of death is first raised by the patient, reflection of his concerns (content and feelings), questions about what conclusions he may have come to, and clarifications of alternative ways of finding the answers are usually more helpful than answering a question directly. Such responses also take the nurse off the spot of being the one who confirms a terminal diagnosis.

  Some patients, however, want to hear the diagnosis first from a nurse as a preliminary sounding board before getting courage to ask the doctor. They then say, "I knew it!"; knowing ahead of time can be a form of control for them. However, even in such instances, the nurses can give tentative or less specific answers such as "Yes, it does look serious," or "It certainly seems like your suspicions of cancer are true." Such less specific answers allow patients to use whatever defenses are necessary to interpret the response. Probably the best response at these times is, "I can't tell you anymore than you already know. It sounds like you need to talk with your physician." Be prepared for silence or excuses. Just listen. Repeat more quietly if they push.
- Find out to whom the patient will talk and encourage time with that person. Notice how the patient feels after certain visitors. Saying, "You seem more (tired, calm, energetic) after (Mary) comes," may help him to become aware of who is helpful to him.
- When the patient voices concerns of dependency, loss, despair, or anxiety, help him to express these feelings rather than quickly reassuring him. Reassurance often feels like discounting the feelings, and the patient may either withdraw and become depressed, feeling no one understands, or act out, complain, or develop somatic difficulties that will be taken seriously.
- Communication with children or young people can be of great comfort and encouragement. Look for ways to arrange it. In the last days of life visits may change to stories, pictures, or relayed messages.
- Encourage the patient who has feelings of guilt, questions about what comes after death, or other spiritual concerns to talk with a chaplain or his minister and arrange it if necessary. Any patient who gives evidence of a religious belief or inner spiritual resources needs to practice his

religion and express and utilize his faith. Questioning a patient who is reticent about speaking of spiritual beliefs may elicit private beliefs that get stronger when expressed or may even uncover vestiges of old beliefs not discarded, but not recently active.

- Prepare family members to expect regression, but encourage them to treat the patient as capable of making decisions and hearing the concerns of family members.
- With the initial diagnosis, patients usually deny and get quiet or have a great need to talk and find out everything they can about the illness and prognosis; the latter response is more common, although it can be masked by denial. Gently asking patients to describe what has been said and how the experience proceeded may help bring them out of the initial shock without pushing for all the feelings and thoughts that will come later. Encourage family members to follow these leads.
- Let the patient relive past or present regrets in his dying.
- Encourage the patient to give or leave special messages about life or memories to "survivors."
- Ask about dreams and fantasies and determine with the patient what meaning these have and if they suggest tasks to be completed or indicate that grieving is being done.
- Have the patient engage with others in a "life review." Sharing memories and perceptions of an experience, as well as chronologically going through one's life, can be a pleasant ending activity. Closing the book on one's life is not easy, but if it is seen as the next chapter and it seems fitting, it may be easier.
- Family members may need reassurance that they are doing all that can be done. Daily information early in the morning concerning the way the patient spent the night helps calm the family and assuage guilt feelings about not being there to watch over him. Letting family know quickly of changes in the patient's condition helps them to develop trust in the nursing care.
- Watch for symbolic or nonverbal language as the patient begins to express fears or wonderings about dying.
- Help family members who have reached a sense of acceptance of the patient's approaching death and who have begun to exclude the patient in decision making and interactions to realize that the patient is not dead yet and needs to be included and not isolated. This is true even if the patient is in a coma.

- If the family wants to keep the diagnosis or prognosis from the patient, and the patient lets the nursing staff know by clues or statements that he is aware, explore with the family members the strengths and weaknesses of the patient and what they fantasize would happen if the patient were told. Then share with them the behaviors that indicate the patient's need or desire to know.
- Do not forget to use humor. Humor can help deal with even the most traumatic part of the illness that otherwise is unspeakable. Don't force humor in order to cheer up the patient. Humor should be natural and come out of the person or the situation.
- When a patient is denying the seriousness of the illness, ask nonthreatening questions that make the patient think about death as a possibility rather than tearing away the denial directly (e.g., "Is your son able to take over your role in the family business?" or "What do you really feel is going to happen to your . . . ?").
- Realize that the patient and his family may differ in their need to know details. Do not assume that what has been told to one family member has been communicated to either the patient or other family members. Check it out.

f. Confront fears of the unknown
- Ask the patient what he has been taught about afterlife.
- Ask about experiences he has had when someone was dying or had died.
- Ask what books he has read on the subject.
- Determine whether the fears center around the dying process, the moment of death, or what happens after death.
- Help him discover and clarify what his religion teaches or what his pastor or rabbi believes.

g. Confront fears of abandonment
- This is especially acute if the living have withdrawn or deserted the dying patient before the need for closeness and interactions has diminished for him. Encourage interaction.
- Assure the patient of continued care and availability. Do not promise to be there when he dies, but assure him of going through the last days with him.
- Let the patient know that if it is his desire, someone can be with him as he is dying. The patient will know and can choose to call someone or slip quietly away, whichever is his style.

- If possible, one special staff member on each shift with whom the patient feels most comfortable should be the one to offer the reassurance of her presence and availability.
- Encourage the patient who believes in a personal God to reinforce through prayer, imagery, or visits from clergy, the belief that God's presence will never leave him alone. (For those of Judeo-Christian faith, reciting the 23rd Psalm, with special emphasis on the promise of comfort through "the valley of the shadow of death," can be very reassuring.)

h. Confront fear of pain and/or loss of dignity

- Once the terminal phase has begun and the pain gets stronger, the strongest medication that does not cause the loss of lucidity should be given. Giving pain medication at regular intervals or at intervals controlled by the patient can prevent pain from reaching intolerable levels. If this is not possible, teach the patient relaxation and breathing exercises to be used when he becomes aware that the pain is ready to increase.
- Treat the patient by touch and words as a person of dignity. Explain the necessity and purpose of procedures and decisions. Conduct personal care matter-of-factly when the patient has lost control of bodily functions, and talk with him while the physical care is being given.

i. Confront fear of loss

- Loss of identity—This loss may be felt when the body does not function well. Loss may also be experienced when others change their response to the patient, or he is unable to respond to them in familiar ways. Finding some aspect that is still intact and has meaning is a challenge, and success pays many dividends in sustaining the quality of life.

  Find some activity that has meaning to the patient, family, or institution that can be done by the patient *for* others. As long as a person feels useful, there is reason to live.
- Loss of the future—The realization that plans and dreams, expectations of activities, and stages of life will never be, needs to be expressed and mourned.
- Loss of relationships—Leaving loved ones behind and mourning both lost and unattainable relationships is an important part of dying. Identifying the losses and mourning them can be helpful. Capturing the good

memories of those relationships by telling stories can bring pleasure as well as focusing on the end.

j. Confront specific fears
   - Listen for individual fears peculiar to the patient's meaning of life.
   - Ask if there are any particular concerns. Permission to disclose these can be given by citing an example such as, "You know, we are all afraid to die."
   - Look for ways to alleviate these particular fears. Ask the patient what would help.

k. Encourage hope
   - In the earlier stages of terminal illness, hope for cures, remissions, time, or miracles may be present. As the patient realizes that the end is in sight, hope for relief from pain, hope of longed-for visits, hope for an event in the near future, or hope for strength to complete a task become important in sustaining interest and purpose in living. Listen for events that spark interest and ask about them or reflect the patient's hopes and anticipation.
   - Sometimes hope becomes bargaining, as Kübler-Ross describes. If it is not detrimental to the patient, allow the process of realization to take its course. If the bargain is injurious to the patient or is evidence of decompensating, gently confront the patient's desire to be without the illness.

l. Tasks and activities
   - After the initial diagnosis, there is still time to accomplish important tasks at work or at home. Find out desires never fulfilled or experiences never taken and encourage the patient to do those activities that will bring satisfaction without harming him or the family financially, emotionally, or physically.
   - Planning for family needs after the death can enable the patient to feel that life still goes on and he has a part in it.
   - Ask the patient or family members if a will has been made. (Over half the population dies without making a will.)
   - Discuss with the patient or encourage him to discuss with family members ideas and desires for a funeral or memorial service. Encourage family members to make arrangements before the death actually occurs, when they have more emotional resources to deal with such decisions.

- Some patients may find it helpful to see family and friends for the last time, to say good-bye, to give messages, or to offer to ask for forgiveness.
- Getting ready spiritually for death is important to most people. Recommend that the chaplain or the patient's personal spiritual advisor spend time frequently so that questions, fears, and feelings can be shared and inner spiritual resources strengthened.

C. Interventions for Care-giving Staff

1. Use staff meetings or conversations with trusted confidants to explore the nursing staff's feelings about dying patients who are close in age or occupation to themselves. (Studies have indicated that staff who identify with the patient are likely to stay away from him.)
2. In team meetings and/or reports, determine what the patient has been told by all involved. Share knowledge with others who will be interacting with the patient.
3. Listen for symbolic cues or questions regarding the fatal progression of the illness and share with team members.

D. Evaluation/Expected Outcomes

Effective nursing care can be evaluated by whether or not the patient is left alone more than nonterminal patients. When nursing staff members feel uncomfortable around a dying patient for whom they can provide nothing more than comfort care, the patient is more likely to be left alone. An evaluation of the patient's comfort level—physical, emotional, and spiritual—can give evidence of effective care, although patients all have their own styles.

1. The nurse will:
   a. Be available to listen.
   b. Ask questions to determine concerns, needs, and tasks of the patient and the family members.
   c. Communicate regularly with the family.
   d. Act as a liaison between the physician and the patient and family.
   e. Insure physical and emotional comfort to the extent possible.
   f. Enlist family and spiritual support.
   g. Discover ways to make the patient's remaining time meaningful.
   h. Treat the patient with respect and enhance his personal dignity.
   i. Help the patient retain as much control as possible.

j. Disclose only as much information as the patient is ready to hear.
k. Follow the lead of the patient in enhancing his approach to death.
l. Develop and use support for herself in the attachment to and detachment from dying patients.
m. Feel comfortable in using natural humor.
n. Discover the uniqueness of each patient.

2. The patient will:
   a. Maintain control of pain.
   b. Interact with family, friends, and staff.
   c. Confront and express fears.
   d. Complete preparations to die.
   e. Engage in activities considered "useful" to the patient.
   f. Express feelings in appropriate ways.
   g. Develop and use any desired spiritual support.
   h. Develop and use social support.
   i. Ask questions of physician(s).
   j. Find ways to express individual uniqueness in "living dying."

E. Evaluation for Referral

After discharge from the hospital, patients and families may be referred for followup and support through organizations such as hospices, private counselors, community support groups, and visiting nurses associations.

IV. POTENTIAL NURSING DIAGNOSES

Because terminal illness involves both physiological and psychological processes, almost any nursing diagnosis could be appropriate, depending on the patient's condition. The ones listed below are some of those related to the dying patient's potential emotional needs.

1. Anxiety, related to
   - anticipation of loss
   - unresolved conflicts
   - fear
2. Comfort, altered, related to physiological or emotional pain

3. Communication, impaired verbal, related to
   - alteration in mental status
   - denial
   - lack of trust
   - depression
   - history of poor communication skills
   - withdrawal
   - inability to express feelings
4. Coping, ineffective individual, related to
   - guilt
   - fear
   - mood disturbance
   - impaired judgment
5. Coping, ineffective family: compromised, related to
   - poor interpersonal relationships
   - anger
   - frustration
   - fear
6. Coping, ineffective family: disabling, related to
   - fear
   - inability to express feelings
   - denial
   - physical aspects of patient care
7. Family processes, alterations in, related to
   - role changes
   - loss of a member of the family
   - financial stress
8. Fear (of death or of the unknown), related to
   - loss of control
   - unpredictable future
9. Grieving, anticipatory, related to
   - anticipation of loss
   - fear
   - changes in self-image
10. Grieving, dysfunctional, related to
    - losses
    - guilt
    - anger
    - unresolved conflict

11. Hopelessness, related to
    - perceived loss
    - altered mental and physical function
    - loss of control
    - loneliness
12. Role disturbance, related to change in previous functioning
13. Self-concept, disturbance in, related to
    - impairment or loss of mental and/or physical function
    - *increased dependence on others for care*
14. Self-care deficit, potential for, related to
    - loss of mental and/or physical function
    - increased dependence on others for care
15. Social isolation, related to
    - feelings of worthlessness
    - sense of abandonment
    - withdrawal
16. Spiritual distress, related to
    - unresolved guilt
    - sense of hopelessness and helplessness
    - unresolved anger
    - inability to forgive self or others

V. SUMMARY

The nurse is in a special position to offer guidance and support to the patient through the difficult process of dying. During the illness the care-giver will seek to discover each individual's style and coping behaviors and to enhance his ability to find significance in the last phases of living.

The nurse will not only seek to bring comfort and relieve the patient's suffering and loneliness, but she will also look for ways to help him recall earlier, healthier days and experience again the sense of well-being and self-esteem. Preserving important relationships, reducing conflict and fear, and increasing the quality of life can be accomplished if the patient is treated as a responsible person capable of clear thinking, significant relationships, and purposeful behavior despite physical deterioration.

Caring for dying patients places intense stress on the nurse. She needs to develop ways of coping with her feelings and reducing her own stress through sharing feelings with colleagues, spending adequate time away from the unit, engaging in physical exercise and relaxation, taking lunch time and breaks, participating in creative activities, and attending courses on stress management techniques.

References

Backer, B. A., Hammon, N., and Russell, N. A. (1982). *Death and dying, individuals and institutions.* New York: John Wiley & Sons.
Benton, R. G. (1987). *Death and dying: Principles and practices in patient care.* New York: D. Van Nostrand Co.
Bowers, M. K., Jackson, E. N., Knight, J. A., et al. (1976). *Counseling the dying* (2nd ed.). New York: Jason Aronson.
Kim, M. J., McFarland, G. K., and McLane, A. M. (1984). *Pocket guide to nursing diagnosis.* St. Louis: C. V. Mosby Company.
Quint, J. C. (1967). *The nurse and the dying patient.* New York: Macmillan Co.
Veterans Administration (1972). *Program guide—Nursing service* (G-10, M-2, Part V). Washington, DC: U.S. Government Printing Office.
Wass, H., Berardo, F. M., and Neimeyer, R. A. (1988). *Dying: Facing the facts* (2nd ed.). Washington, DC: Hemisphere Publishing Corporation.
Yeager, C. S. (1983). Coping with loss and aging. In J. Howe, E. J. Dickason, D. A. Jones, et al. (Eds.), *The handbook of nursing.* New York: John Wiley & Sons.

Chapter 18

The Patient with a Spiritual Need

Roberta L. Messner *Doreen Ward*

I. STATEMENT OF PURPOSE

Throughout the many seasons of life—happiness and heartbreak, triumph and tragedy, peacefulness and pain—nurses are there. For each accomplishment and adversity, however, there is an accompanying spiritual dimension—an opportunity to discover deeper meaning and to affirm the profound existence of a higher power.

Nurses interact with patients on a more intimate level than any other health care provider and are frequently the patient's initial resource during a crisis or significant life event. It is therefore no accident that "whys" are often first verbalized and "masks" are initially relinquished within the presence of a caring nurse. For these reasons, addressing a patient's spiritual needs represents both an opportunity and an obligation if holistic nursing care is to be delivered.

The purpose of this chapter is:

- To present a nursing framework for the provision of spiritual support that respects the diversity of individual belief systems, recognizing the nurse as an aide and collaborator with other spiritual resource persons.
- To assist the nurse in more comfortably utilizing the nursing process to promote, maintain, and restore spiritual health and wholeness.

II. OVERVIEW OF SPIRITUALITY

The quest for physical, psychosocial, and spiritual well-being is a universal human pursuit. Spiritual health is related to all aspects of health, influencing the ability to love and be loved and to forgive and be forgiven (Fish and Shelly 1983). Throughout all of life, the spiritual realm—although frequently neglected in basic nursing curriculum, continuing education, administration, and practice—can be an individual's most important stabilizing force and support system.

Stallwood (1975) states that a spiritual need is the absence of any factor necessary to sustain a dynamic, individual relationship with God. Spiritual distress is exhibited when a person views himself as incomplete or inadequate in some aspect of his life (Kreidler 1984). In Pray's (1984) experience, "outgrowing the desire to tell God what 'should have been' made room for a deeper faith. In hindsight, he viewed his inadequacy (secondary to his diabetes) as a card player who spent so much time protesting his hand (his illness) he wasn't getting to the game." He discovered spiritual health when he acknowledged that the phrase "if only" is based on comparisons, and prevents our finding and expressing God's unique creation within each of us.

Spiritual beliefs influence a myriad of lifestyle decisions that ultimately affect physical health such as the acceptance of preventive health modalities, sexual practices, use of alcohol, tobacco, and drugs, and dietary customs. Perhaps even more critical to nursing, however, is that the spiritual dimension unifies the total human experience. The spiritual cry may appear muffled by technology, but is ever-present and real.

III. NURSING MANAGEMENT

Comprehensive nursing management of the individual with a spiritual need includes assessment, planning, intervention, and evaluation. Because the spiritual needs and capacities of children vary with each stage of development, the following discussion is applicable only to the adult patient. The reader is referred to *The Spiritual Needs of Children* (Shelly 1982).

A. Assessment

It is important to realize that healthy religious practices move a person toward health and wholeness. The basis of a spiritual assessment is to plan nursing care that will promote spiritual health. Before initiating a spiritual assessment, the physical and emotional health of the patient should be appraised, since physical and psychiatric crises may involve marked spiritual dysfunction (Braverman 1987) that will preclude immediate, detailed assessment of spiritual needs. Furthermore, patients with alterations in thought processes may exhibit distortions in regard to spirituality, such as delusions involving religious content. Individuals with personality or character disorders may use religion for manipulative purposes.

If a patient with a psychiatric history appears preoccupied with religious thoughts or rituals, it is important to thoroughly assess if this is a recent or long-standing interest; circumstances surrounding the patient's introduction to the ideas; relationship of the ideas to the patient's background and familial values; and any relationship between the patient's religious concerns and psychiatric behavior (John 1983).

A complete spiritual assessment should be incorporated into the initial nursing assessment. This provides essential direction for all apsects of care and provides valuable insight into the patient's response to illness and treatment. Freedom of religion does not have to mean freedom from religion; in fact, some institutions include a spiritual assessment as part of the initial data base. Nonetheless, because of the highly personalized nature of spirituality, this assessment should be reserved for the latter part of the interview, after rapport has been established. Patients may be puzzled by the spiritual aspect of the nursing history. If so, simply explain the rationale for knowing the patient's sources of strength to enhance his care. Stoll (1979) suggests structuring the assessment as follows:

1. What is the patient's concept of his God? Does he acknowledge the presence of a divine source in his life? If so, how does he describe this presence and how important is it to him?
2. What is the patient's source of hope, comfort, and strength? Who does he turn to in times of joy, stress, aloneness, and crisis?
3. What religious rituals/practices are important to the patient? What are his patterns of worship?
4. Does the patient see any relationship between his spiritual beliefs and his health or current life situation? Does he feel that his faith is being challenged by a current event in his life?

   The following aspects of assessment, as described by Fish and Shelly (1983), are important to determine initially as well as on an ongoing basis to indicate the possibility of a spiritual need.

5. What is the patient's affect and attitude? Does he appear despondent, isolated, angry, guilty, anxious, hopeless, powerless, preoccupied, or struggling with inner conflicts?

6. What is the patient's behavior? Does he give thanks before meals, pray at bedtime, or read religious materials?
7. Does the patient talk about his faith or his church? Verbalizations of religious clichés do not assure spiritual health and may even signal inner conflict. Likewise, use of profanity or joking about spiritual issues does not necessarily indicate the patient is not concerned with spiritual issues. What are the patient's defense mechanisms? Do they mask an underlying spiritual need?
8. What is the content and quality of the patient's interpersonal relationships? How does the patient interact with family, friends, clergy, and staff?
9. Assess the patient's environment. Does the patient have a Bible, religious medals, or greeting cards with religious messages? Such belongings may provide clues to the patient's concerns or the concerns of his significant others. Does the patient listen to inspirational music on the radio or view religious programs on television?
10. How does the patient see the role of the nurse in supporting his spiritual concerns? Would he like his pastor, the hospital chaplain, or any other individual to be notified of his hospitalization?
11. Does the patient have any sensory or mobility disturbances? This will affect planning of spiritual care (reading versus listening to the radio or to tapes, the ability to attend chapel services, and so on).

In summary, a spiritual assessment includes an appraisal of spiritual coping strategies. Activities utilized by patients may include personal prayer or asking others to pray with them; reading the Bible or inspirational books; listening to religious television, radio, or music; or possession of objects such as plaques, rosaries, and wall hangings. Spiritual endeavors during periods of stress can be viewed as one kind of direct coping action. Lazarus (1980) emphasizes that patients experiencing life-threatening illnesses often rely on faith for hope and comfort while coping. Hence, religious faith is a coping strategy that may lessen the negative impact of illness and provide stability during any life-change event.

When assessing the spiritual realm, remember that any change in one's spiritual need is also a stressor that may require intervention. Interestingly, the Holmes-Rahe Social Readjustment Rating Scale lists "change in church activities" (a lot more or less than usual) as a life-change event that is accompanied by stress (Reale 1987).

B. Planning

Planning of nursing interventions is based on the aforementioned nursing assessment and the formulation of appropriate nursing diagnoses. Planning of care in response to an identified spiritual need should be a joint effort between the nurse and patient, and founded on the patient's unique spiritual belief system. But before you begin to plan, honestly examine your own spiritual beliefs. This can help you to advise your patient in the plan that will most meet his needs.

C. Intervention

1. Prevention

   Early recognition of spiritual needs and the prevention of spiritual distress or a spiritual crisis is dependent on a careful ongoing nursing assessment, as previously outlined, and carefully planned, individualized intervention.
2. Treatment

   Swindoll (1983) emphasizes that the persons who are most influential in our lives are those individuals who exemplify the attributes of consistency, authenticity, unselfishness, and tirelessness. These characteristics constitute the core of spiritual care.
   a. *Consistency*. Be dependable in your approach to the patient. Do not make promises you are unable to fulfill. This is the foundation of trust in the nurse-patient relationship. Provide a consistent environment for the patient by helping him carry out religious practices that provide strength, comfort, and hope.
   b. *Authenticity*. Do not pretend to be someone you are not. Even individuals with a similar religious framework may have differences of opinions in values and beliefs. It is not necessary to agree with a patient's spiritual convictions to support and help him.
   c. *Unselfishness*. Base spiritual care on the patient's identified needs, not yours.
   d. *Tirelessness*. Help the patient to procure resources necessary to practice religious beliefs (with appropriate administrative approval). Be attentive to details.
3. Medications

   The nursing process may reveal that for a particular

individual, spiritual rather than medical intervention is most appropriate in selected circumstances. When this is determined, reading of Biblical passages and/or prayer may, for example, be more effective than a sedative. This interdisciplinary decision should be communicated on the nursing care plan as well as to other members of the multidisciplinary team. Consider, for example, a patient who has had a lens implant. He is accustomed to reading his Bible every night but now his vision is impaired. He complains of insomnia during his stay. A caring nurse responds to his expressed need by reading a favorite scripture to him. Subsequent evaluation of this intervention reveals that the patient had a restful night.

4. Nursing Actions

   It is beyond the scope of this chapter to include all nursing interventions for the individual manifesting a spiritual need. Each person's spiritual frame of reference is highly personal, and interventions should be based on prior establishment of rapport and trust, a comprehensive nursing assessment, provisions for privacy, and appropriate timing of interventions. Some possible interventions are as follows.

   a. Assess the significance of spirituality to the patient.
   b. Listen to the patient with your heart as well as your mind, providing an atmosphere conducive to sharing of memories, present concerns, and future dreams. Be attuned to subtle expressions of spiritual concerns.
   c. Affirm the patient's unique worth and dignity as a human being as well as his observed strengths in coping with illness and other significant life events. This is accomplished both verbally and nonverbally. Consider, for example, a patient with AIDS who states, "No one cares. I'm not even worth the hospital bed space." The nurse and patient could explore feelings that may serve as barriers to tapping spiritual and human resources in order to help the patient discover meaningful purpose.
   d. Encourage dialogue that clarifies and refines spiritual beliefs and explores past experiences that have rendered strength and affirmed the faithfulness of the patient's God. Give the patient an opportunity to express his source of faith and hope in life's circumstances, as well as spiritual aspects for his treatment regimen. Do not pursue trivial issues, but focus on what is important to the patient, using the patient's terminology, in an atmosphere of privacy.
   e. Acknowledge that every step in the coping process—denial, anger, depression, bargaining, and acceptance—has an accompanying spiritual component. Assess the patient's be-

havior and defense mechanisms to guide nursing interventions.

f. Establish a collaborative relationship with hospital chaplains and local clergy. Relate to the patient's clergy—his *primary* spiritual resource—any pertinent information about the patient's health or behavior. This information serves to prepare the clergy for the patient's state of physical or emotional distress, enabling him to deal effectively with the patient's concerns without restraint or hesitancy. If a patient's physical appearance is altered by wires, tubes, or edema, and a portrayal of such is known beforehand, the initial approach can be less alarming and uneasy. If a stroke has rendered an individual aphasic, the clergy will be prepared to expect altered means of communication.

   Should a patient's desire or request be made known to you, try to meet that need if feasible. This mutual sharing of information will help each discipline to better understand complementary roles and the ultimate relationship between physical, psychosocial, and spiritual health.

   A nurse's experience and training in matters of spiritual health generally is limited, so feelings of inadequacy may not be uncommon. Sometimes being a sensible and caring listener may not be enough. The most powerful resource for the patient experiencing spiritual distress may be his clergy or hospital chaplain, an individual who is trained in the spiritual guidance that can lead to spiritual peace and understanding. The clergy should be acknowledged as a valued member of the health care team—a "physician" for the soul.

g. Inform the patient of religious services provided by your institution. If the patient is not ambulatory, arrange transportation to and from the service. Ask the patient if he wishes to be visited by the chaplain or another member of the clergy and initiate appropriate referrals. Prepare for these visits by refreshing and dressing the patient. Provide privacy and an uncluttered, neat environment during these visits, so the patient will feel free to discuss religious concerns openly. Offer to assist with bedside spiritual observances or in arranging certain religious rituals as needed.

h. Query the patient as to his personal religious customs so that they may be supported, if possible, during the hospitalization. Virtually all faiths have accompanying practices, rituals, or holy laws. Should the patient's religious belief prohibit him from participating in a medical treatment regimen, make sure the ramifications are made known to him. In your role as nurse-counselor, you are responsible for providing all the information the patient needs in order to make a knowledgeable decision, while maintaining a nonjudgmental atmosphere.

i. Help the patient obtain desired religious materials that provide comfort, including the preferred Biblical translation, if feasible. If a Jewish male wears a yarmulke, it should not be removed if at all possible.

j. The scriptures provide a discussion of every human need and emotion. Judicious selection and reading of Biblical passages that parallel the patient's circumstances may render strength and comfort. Reading of scripture or other religious materials should be in response to the patient's expressed desires and should never be recited in an attempt to exert control or, as a general rule, with patients who have disturbances in thought processes. Be sensitive to the patient's cues. Attempts at spiritual support without some indication of the patient's desires will only serve to create undue anxiety.

k. Prayer is a practice common to all faiths. Through prayer, God—however defined by the patient—is characterized as available and accessible. It is acceptable for the nurse to pray with a patient (silently or audibly) if the patient requests it. Prayer may be extemporaneous or structured, but should reflect a thorough nursing assessment and the patient's concerns, not the nurse's. The patient's actual words can be used to compose a brief, simple prayer, or a prayer with special meaning for the patient (such as the Lord's Prayer) may be recited. Joint prayer with a patient not only establishes communication with his God, but strengthens a human connection as well. Looking to a divine source can render meaning when earthly resources have been exhausted. Prayer, however, should never be used to strip the patient of his defenses, to pressure the patient to discuss intimate issues he wishes to remain private (Conrad 1985), or to reinforce delusions or unrealistic expectations.

l. If you are not comfortable discussing spiritual concerns (in particular, emotionally charged topics such as divine healing and various spiritual gifts) with a patient who has an identified spiritual need, initiate a referral to the chaplain, pastor, or another staff member who is comfortable with the situation and has established a rapport with the patient.

D. Evaluation/Expected Outcomes

Effective nursing management will be evaluated in terms of the patient's response to the individualized interventions encompassing spiritual care. This involves a delicate balance between the nurse's values and beliefs and the patient's needs. Many nurses view their profession as a "calling," and those with strong religious convictions may feel compelled to try to convert an individual to their own belief systems. The key is to meet the patient's needs, not the care-giver's. Understand that different religions have different rituals, language, and customs. Do not impose your own prayers or rituals.

The patient experiencing spiritual pain needs understanding and support, not preaching or attempts to convert him. Any pressure to explore unfamiliar spiritual values can only add to the already heavy burden of spiritual distress and result in guilt, anxiety, and disruption of care. Implore the patient to help you understand how you can be of assistance.

1. The nurse will incorporate spiritual care into ongoing patient care by assisting the patient to articulate spiritual concerns and to find purpose and significance in illness and other significant life events in the context of the patient's spiritual belief system.
2. The patient will maintain or improve spiritual health by finding a purpose and meaning in illness and other significant life events and by participation in spiritual practices that do not conflict with the treatment plan.

E. Evaluation for Referral

Spiritual distress may be verbalized or expressed indirectly through anger, depression, or fear. It is an astute and sensitive nurse who can trace these elements back to spirituality and then verify the patient's need in this area through a nursing assessment.

Once the importance of spirituality is established, find out if the patient wants to talk with someone. Clarify the patient's choice of counselor, whether it be his own pastor, the hospital chaplain, or another nurse or individual who is comfortable with the subject. Sometimes a patient is more open and at ease revealing his troubled spirit to someone who does not "know" him.

If the patient has no faith, determine what has sustained him during difficult times and reinforce those things. For example, if the patient has a love of music and it has helped him over life's humps in the past, it can be used to lift his spirits now. Let the patient know that you are there and ready to help.

IV. POTENTIAL NURSING DIAGNOSES

Because spiritual needs are a part of virtually every human experience, potential nursing diagnoses related to spirituality are numerous. The reader is referred to the publications on nursing diagnoses and to Carson (1989). At present only one nursing diagnosis specifically addresses the spiritual component of patient care (Kim et al. 1984):

1. Spiritual distress, related to
   - separation from religious/cultural ties as evidenced by anxiety, insomnia, guilt, questioning the meaning of life's events
   - unresolved guilt or anger
   - feelings of powerlessness

V. SUMMARY

Spiritual health is "the affirmation of life in a relationship with God, self, community, and environment that nutures and celebrates wholeness" (White House Conference on Aging 1971). Although for a number of reasons, spiritual care is frequently overlooked by nurses, research shows that patients indeed look to nurses with their spiritual concerns.

Illness and other significant life events challenge spiritual values and should be addressed in the context of the nurse-patient relationship. There are many potential resources for meeting a patient's spiritual needs: religious rituals, referrals to clergy, prayer, and reading of scripture. However, the most important resource for nursing is the powerful instrument of self, which integrates compassion, understanding, and a keen sensitivity to individual values and belief systems.

References

Braverman, E. R. (1987). The religious medical model: Holy medicine and the spiritual behavior inventory. *Southern Medical Journal, 80*(4), 415–420.

Campbell, C. (1984). *Nursing diagnosis and intervention in nursing practice* (2nd ed.). New York: John Wiley & Sons.

Carson, V. B. (1989). *Spiritual dimensions of nursing practice.* Philadelphia: W. B. Saunders.

Conrad, N. L. (1985). Spiritual support for the dying. *Nursing Clinics of North America, 20*(2), 415–425.

Fish, S., and Shelly, J. A. (1983). *Spiritual care—The nurse's role* (2nd ed.). Downers Grove, IL: Inter Varsity Press.

Ferszt, G. G., and Taylor, P. B. (1988). When your patient needs spiritual comfort. *Nursing 88, 18*(4), 48–49.

John, S. D. (1983). Assessing spiritual needs. In J. A. Shelly et al. (Eds.), *Spiritual Dimensions of Mental Health.* Downers Grove, IL: Inter Varsity Press.

Kim, M. J., McFarland, G. K., and McLane, A. M. (1984). *Pocket guide to nursing diagnoses.* St. Louis: C. V. Mosby Co.

Kreidler, M. (1984). Meaning in suffering. *International Nursing Review, 31*(6), 174–76.

Lazarus, R. S. (1980). The stress and coping paradigm. In L. Bonde and J. C. Rosen (Eds.), *Competence and coping during adulthood.* Hanover, NH: University Press of New England, pp. 28–69.

Pray, L. (1984). When disease strikes. *Your Life and Health,* August, 22–23.

Reale, J. (1987). Life changes: Can they cause disease? *Nursing 87, 17*(7), 52–55.

Shelly, J. A. (1982). *The spiritual needs of children.* Downers Grove, IL: Inter Varsity Press.

Stallwood, J. (1975). Spiritual dimensions of nursing practice. In I. Belard and J. Passos (Eds.), *Clinical nursing* (3rd ed.). New York: Macmillan.

Stoll, R. J. (1979). Guidelines for spiritual assessment. *American Journal of Nursing, 79*(9), 1574–1577.

Swindoll, C. R. (1983). *Growing strong in the seasons of life.* Portland, OR: Multnomah Press.

White House Conference on Aging. (1971). *Spiritual well-being.* Washington, DC: U.S. Government Printing Office, p. 1.

Chapter 19

The Family of the Hospitalized Patient

Jo Annalee Irving

I. STATEMENT OF PURPOSE

The entire family— not just the patient—experiences the stresses associated with a family member being hospitalized. A hospitalization often produces anxiety and unanticipated difficulties for the family system.

The purpose of this chapter is:

- To increase the nurse's understanding of the response of family members to a hospitalized family member.
- To facilitate nursing management of family members who are potentially or actively involved in the hospitalization experience of an ill family member.

II. OVERVIEW OF THE FAMILY OF THE HOSPITALIZED PATIENT

A. Description of the Behavior

When a family member is hospitalized, both the patient and the family face a number of adaptive tasks. Pre-established rules and roles in the family may have to change to accommodate the needs of the entire family system.

B. Incidence

It is predictable that family members or significant others will be present when an illness requires an individual to be hospitalized. How often and how many people will visit may be determined, to some extent, by the visiting policies of the hospital. In addition, past interpersonal relationships and physical distance will also determine who visits. It is important for the nurse to have a broad perspective of the definition of family. Individuals who are important to the patient may defy the traditional definition of family (that is, two or more persons who are joined by marriage, blood, or adoption and who interact with one another but may not live together). In order for the nurse to incorporate visitors selectively in the patient's care, a flexible conceptualization of family enhances utilization of those important people in the patient's life. The hospital setting can lessen or deprive both the family and the patient of the psychological and emotional support they experience at home. In addition, the particular disease process of the ill family member can adversely affect the physical and emotional separation of the family (e.g., stroke or coma).

In an effort to maintain homeostasis, the family's reaction to disequilibrium may be dealt with through a temporary or permanent redefinition of itself. There are many stressors potentially at play for the patient and the family during the crisis of hospitalization.

C. Clinical Manifestations

The hospitalization of a family member can be an anxiety-producing experience at the least for some families and a crisis situation for others. A myriad of variables will determine the family's response. The following are not inclusive, but potential responses manifested by family members include:

anxiety; hostility; depression; blame; guilt; restlessness; hyperactivity; tearfulness; crying; loneliness; demands; anger; fear; powerlessness; tension; poor concentration; loss of appetite; verbal abuse; impaired decision making; role strain; role overload; financial concerns; criticism of nursing care; cultural shock (the hospital environment); passive-aggressive behavior; overfunctioning or underfunctioning; conflict among family members; withdrawal from the patient or other family members; minimizing a serious or critical situation; use of repetition with staff to avoid facing threatening issues; inappropriate use of humor.

III. NURSING MANAGEMENT

The realities of the clinical setting, such as work load, time factors, staffing, and activity levels of patients, all interfere with the amount of involvement nurses are able to have with family members.

A. Assessment

The process of family involvement begins with the patient on admission. It is here that the first opportunities arise to assess the patient's needs in the context of the family. If the family is not interviewed on admission, the nursing staff will have to create other opportunities to communicate with family and significant others when they visit the patient.

Assessment questions the nurse might consider asking the patient, family members, and significant others are:

1. Who will be visiting the patient while he is in the hospital?
2. Are there family members or others the patient does not wish to have as visitors in the hospital?
3. What are the expectations of the family/significant others about visiting the ill family member?
4. Are there family members or others who cannot visit because of distance or obligations with whom the patient would like contact?
5. What are the ethnic, racial, or religious backgrounds that may influence family interaction as well as participation in patient care?
6. What is the family's past experience with the hospitalization of a family member?
7. What are the family members' current expectations about the ill family member?
8. What is the patient's expectation about the family being involved in his care?
9. What family members are willing to participate in the patient's care?
10. What are the expectations of the family regarding the nursing staff?
11. What role changes, if any, will occur for the hospitalized patient?
12. What resources need to be mobilized to facilitate those role changes?
13. Who is a designated spokesperson or leader in the family?
14. Does the family have an identified support system outside the family?
15. What is the most important concern of the patient about his family?
16. What is the most important concern of the family about the patient?

The interview also provides the opportunity to observe and assess the interaction among patient, family, and significant others present.

B. Planning

The planning of nursing care for the family or significant others of the hospitalized patient will be based on the ongoing assessment during the hospitalized patient's stay. It will be most beneficial to the patient, family, and nursing staff if planning is done with the patient's and family's needs in mind and is not based on the timing of services that are most convenient to the nurse.

Patient care is thus ultimately planned with the total family in mind. Families that are fully aware of the care plan are in a better position to support each other and the patient.

C. Intervention

1. Prevention

   Most hospitalized patients will have family or significant others visiting during their hospital stay. There is no accumulated evidence that can assist in the prediction of the family's and others' response to the hospitalized patient. While nursing staff cannot be expected to be family therapists, they cannot afford to overlook the distinctions between the patient's needs and the family's needs during this period. The best precautions for staying in touch with these needs lies in the initial and ongoing assessment process, as well as in the utilization of other hospital resources such as the psychiatric nurse, nurse clinical specialist, or social worker.

2. Treatment

   In hospitals that consider themselves family-centered health care institutions, a climate for supportive family services will usually pre-exist. These hospitals will provide educational programs for staff to prepare them to include families along with the patient in the plan of care. The major focus is on the relationship between personnel, patients, and the family.

   When these programs do not pre-exist, the recognition of the family's needs and responses to a hospitalized family member will depend on the individual nurse and how those needs are considered in the plan of care.

3. Medications

   During the initial assessment and/or the ongoing assessment process, the knowledge of medications being taken and any physical disabilities of family members would assist the nurse in the physical, emotional, and cognitive evaluation of the family constellation. Because the hospitalization period is a stressful time for the family, additional reactions to taking medications can arise. In addition, the family member(s) may have need for medications for symptoms of stress, anxiety, and sleeplessness, as well as other needs.

4. Nursing Actions
   a. Acknowledge to the family that the nurse is aware that this is a most stressful time.

b. Assist in decreasing the family's fear and promote a sense of control by providing simple descriptions and explanations.
c. Provide general information about the hospitalization period and what the usual progression of events are.
d. If hospital-based support exists, link the family when it is appropriate.
e. Recognize family strengths; identify and affirm coping strategies they have used in the past that were successful.
f. Recognize the differences between cognitive requests (information seeking) and emotional requests (expressing feelings or needing support) from family members.
g. When family dynamics are continuously conflictual or destructive, involve an appropriate consultant.
h. Recognize that some family members will have difficulty in any care-giving roles. Support their decision not to participate.
i. Recognize that family members may be able to diminish their anxiety when they are included in the patient's care.
j. Contract with the family a mutual care agreement so your relationship becomes collaborative rather than competitive. For example, the nursing staff and family will divide assisting Mr. H. with his four walks down the hall; the nursing staff will assist Mrs. W. with breakfast and supper and Mrs. W.'s family will assist her with lunch.
k. Encourage expression of feelings without judgment.
l. Recognize that other family dynamics may coexist when distant family members convene together in the hospital.
m. Provide for privacy for family members to vent their emotions or cry.
n. When there are many family members, have them identify a family spokesperson.
o. In some instances it may be helpful to have one or two nurses be the family's liaison to the hospital staff.
p. Provide outlets for the nurse who deals with unusual stress from a family (e.g., rotate the staff, let nurse vent her feelings, and enlist consultation from a clinical specialist or social worker).
q. Set limits with overbearing family members who threaten the progress of the patient.
r. Discuss family expectations.
s. Give family members who need it permission to leave the hospital in order to have some personal time away.
t. Continue ongoing observations and assessments of family members during the hospitalization period.

D. Evaluation/Expected Outcomes

Nursing management can be evaluated in terms of observed family behaviors.

The family will:

1. Have an orientation to the hospital environment and routines that affect the patient.
2. Be able to express fears and concerns about the hospitalization experience.
3. Understand the nursing plan of care for the patient.
4. Be able to communicate with each other as well as to the patient about the given illness.
5. Be selectively involved in the patient's care as they feel comfortable and as it is an appropriate part of the nursing plan.
6. Be referred to appropriate resources when their behavior or needs are out of the realm of the nurse's background.
7. Be able to manage their visitor roles and maintain constructive roles at home.
8. Not jeopardize their own physical or emotional health due to feelings of obligation to the hospitalized family member.
9. Rely on other outside resources when necessary.
10. Engage in sound problem-solving processes.

E. Evaluation for Referral

In family situations within the hospital in which the staff nurse cannot effectively intervene, either because of time restraints or insufficient background in family dynamics, in-house resources can be solicited. The psychiatric nurse clinical specialist, social worker, or perhaps somconc from pastoral counseling are all possibilities for first-line resources. Any of these individuals could do further assessment of the family situation and make an appropriate disposition.

If these services are immediately available within the hospital, then the appropriate channels within nursing service should be followed for problems that are on the staff nurses' level. The hospitalized family member's physician might be consulted about the family. The family's minister or rabbi, if appropriate, might be another resource. The local community mental health center might be contacted for family services; selected self-help groups in the community might be another resource, depending on the nature of the issues (e.g., an Alzheimer's family support group, mastectomy group, or hospice). Other community agencies such as the American Cancer Society and the American Heart Association may be links to support for families. The most important aspects of the nurse's role with these families are to listen, to be nonjudgmental, and to link with other resources. (*Note*: Occasionally a family continues to be problematic to staff even after emotional support and other resources are given. In such an instance, limits must be established in order to prevent jeopardizing the care of the hospitalized family member or other patients on the unit. In select cases hospital administration and/or hospital security may need to be involved.)

IV. POTENTIAL NURSING DIAGNOSES

1. Family process, alterations in, related to
   - illness of family member
   - discomforts associated with the symptoms of illness
   - change in family members' ability to function
   - separation
   - hospitalization
   - loss of body part or function
   - expensive treatments
   - disabling treatments
   - surgery
   - time-consuming treatments
   - inability to accept or receive help appropriately
   - inability to adapt to change or to deal with traumatic experiences constructively
   - inability to express or accept wide range of feelings/feelings of members
   - rigidity in function and roles
   - ineffective family decision-making process
   - failure to send and receive clear messages
   - unexamined family myths
   - inappropriate boundary maintenance
   - inappropriate or poorly communicated family rules, rituals, symbols.

V. SUMMARY

This chapter has highlighted some of the activities the staff nurse might encounter when dealing with the family of a hospitalized patient. Clearly, the nurse's awareness of the family's emotional reactions and needs can present an added responsibility to the nursing care of patients. However, through cogent family assessment the nurse can gain valuable data about the family system and enhance the nursing of the family member, as well as intervening into stressful responses of the family.

References

Carpenito, L. J. (1987). *Nursing diagnosis: Application to clinical practice.* Philadelphia: J. B. Lippincott Company.

Doenges, M. E., and Modyhouse, M. F. (1985). *Nurses pocket guide: Nursing diagnoses with interventions.* Philadelphia: F. A. Davis Company.

Duvall, E. M. (1972). *Marriage and family development.* Philadelphia: J. B. Lippincott Company.

Friedman, M. L., and Tubergen, P. (1987). Multiple sclerosis and the family. *Archives of Psychiatric Nursing, (1),* 47–54.

McCubbin, H. I. (1979). Integrating coping behavior in family stress theory. *Journal of Marriage and the Family, 2,* 237–244.

Meleis, A. I., and Swendsen, L. A. (1978). Role supplementation: An empirical test of a nursing intervention. *Nursing Research, 27,* 11–18.

Miller, S., and Winstead-Fry, P. (1982). *Family systems theory in nursing practice.* Virginia: Reston Publishing Company.

Mishel, M. H., and Murdaugh, C. L. (1987). Family adjustment to heart transplantation: Redesigning the dream. *Nursing Research, 36,* 332–338.

Moos, R. (1977). The crisis of physical illness–An overview. In R. Moos (Ed.), *Coping with physical illness.* New York: Plenum Publishing Company.

Turks, D. C., and Kems, R. D. (1985). *Health, illness and families.* New York: John Wiley & Sons.

Welch, D. (1981). Planning nursing interventions for family members of adult cancer patients. *Cancer Nursing, 15,* 365–370.

SECTION FIVE

OTHER ISSUES

Chapter 20

Psychotropic Medications

Theodore B. Feldmann

I. STATEMENT OF PURPOSE

The advent of psychotropic medications, drugs that exert various direct effects on the central nervous system to modify pathological behavior, has revolutionized the treatment of psychiatric disorders. With these drugs, even the most severe psychiatric symptoms can be controlled to a certain extent, leading to shorter hospital stays, an emphasis on outpatient treatment, and an overall improvement in the level of functioning for the affected individual. Advances in neurochemistry and neurophysiology have also shed considerable light on the pathogenesis of psychiatric disorders.

This chapter is designed to provide the nurse with a basic introduction to psychotropic medications. Each of the major groups of drugs will be presented, with emphasis on the mechanism of action, indications and contraindications for use, side effects, and dose ranges.

II. ANTIPSYCHOTIC DRUGS

The antipsychotic drugs, formerly referred to as major tranquilizers, are now called neuroleptics. This group consists of a number of different agents that differ mainly in their potency and side effect profiles. The antipsychotic drugs directly effect disturbances of thought and perception, control agitated and disturbed behavior, and produce varying degrees of sedation. All the members of this group have the potential for annoying, and sometimes serious, side effects. As a group, however, they have little or no potential for abuse or addiction.

A. Mechanism of Action

1. All drugs in this group affect the central neurotransmitter dopamine. The drugs act to block dopamine receptors, creating in effect a functional deficiency of the neurotransmitter.

2. Dopamine has been shown to be important in the development of schizophrenic symptoms. Psychomotor stimulants, such as amphetamines, are powerful releasers of dopamine. Administration of high doses of amphetamines produces a paranoid psychosis very similar to paranoid schizophrenia. The therapeutic action of the antipsychotics, therefore, appears to be related to the ability to block the dopamine receptors.
3. Dopamine also plays a role in regulating movement. It has been shown, for example, that patients with Parkinson's disease have a deficiency of dopamine. This fact is important in understanding the parkinsonian side effects of the antipsychotic drugs.

B. Indications

1. The primary indication for this group of drugs is the presence of a psychosis.
2. Target symptoms of the antipsychotic drugs include:
   a. Hallucinations
   b. Delusions
   c. Thought disorder
   d. Inappropriate affect
   e. Disturbed psychomotor behavior (e.g., catatonia)
   f. Agitation
3. Specific disorders in which these drugs are useful include:
   a. Schizophrenia
   b. Mania
   c. Psychotic depression
   d. Psychosis associated with organic brain syndromes
   e. Conditions accompanied by extreme degrees of agitation

C. Side Effects and Toxicity

1. There are no absolute contraindications for the use of the antipsychotic drugs.
2. Autonomic side effects are frequently encountered and are due to the drugs' anticholinergic and antiadrenergic properties. These side effects include dry mouth, blurred vision, constipation, urinary retention, paralytic ileus, confusion, miosis or mydriasis, and postural hypotension.

   Side effects usually improve with a reduction of the antipsychotic dose.
3. The central anticholinergic syndrome may occur in patients taking antipsychotic medications with strong anticholinergic properties. It consists of agitation, confusion, high fever, hallucinations, dilated pupils, and seizures. Stupor and coma may

follow. Treatment consists of discontinuing the medication and administering physostigmine, 2 mg IV, which may be repeated every hour as necessary.

4. Neuroleptic malignant syndrome is a rare but potentially fatal side effect whose cause is unknown. It has a mortality of up to 20%. The signs and symptoms include hyperthermia, muscle rigidity, confusion and disorientation, respiratory distress, labile blood pressure, and eventually cardiovascular collapse. Treatment consists of the immediate discontinuation of all antipsychotic medications and supportive care.
5. Extrapyramidal side effects
   a. Dystonias consist of bizarre movements of the tongue, face, and neck. These reactions, which are extremely frightening to the patient, include torticollis, oculogyric crisis, and opisthotonos. Treatment consists of benztropine (Cogentin), 2 mg IV or IM; biperiden (Akineton), 2 mg IM; or trihexyphenidl (Artane), 5 mg IM or PO. These are antiparkinsonian drugs, which have powerful anticholinergic effects. Diazepam (Valium) may be given 10 mg IV, as well as diphenhydramine (Benadryl), 50 mg IV. Oral benztropine (Cogentin) or trihexyphenidl (Artane) may be used prophylactically, at a dose of 2 mg up to three times a day.
   b. Akathisia is a distressing side effect marked by feelings of motor restlessness in which the patient feels the constant urge to move around and has great difficulty sitting still. Treatment with benztropine often controls this symptom.
   c. Parkinsonian effects consist of rigidity, masked facies, resting tremor, shuffling gait, and psychomotor retardation. This side effect responds readily to benztropine.
   d. Tardive dyskinesia is a late-appearing extrapyramidal side effect consisting of chronic buccofacialmandibular or buccolingual movements, and choreoathetoid movements of the extremities. It is thought to result from an increase in dopamine synthesis and receptor supersensitivity in response to prolonged dopamine blockade. There is no specific treatment, and discontinuation or dose reduction of the drug is recommended.
6. Other side effects include:
   a. Cholestatic jaundice
   b. Agranulocytosis
   c. Skin and eye photosensitivity
   d. Lowering of the seizure threshold
   e. Breast engorgement and lactation in female patients
   f. Delayed ejaculation or impotence in males

g. Retinitis pigmentosa with doses of thioridazine in excess of 800 mg/day

D. Specific Agents (see Table 20–1 for dose ranges)

1. Phenothiazines
   a. Chlorpromazine (Thorazine) and thioridazine (Mellaril) are high-dose, low-potency agents. Both have a high degree of sedation and strong anticholinergic properties.
   b. Fluphenazine (Prolixin), perphenazine (Trilafon), and trifluoperazine (Stelazine) are low-dose, high-potency agents. These drugs produce less sedation, but have a higher incidence of extrapyramidal side effects.
2. Butyrophenones: haloperidol (Haldol) is the only representative of this group in clinical use. It is a low-dose, high-potency agent, which has very little sedation. It tends to have a high incidence of extrapyramidal side effects.
3. Thioxanthenes: thiothixene (Navane) is very similar to haloperidol.
4. Dibenzoxazepines: loxapine (Loxitane) is somewhat more sedating than haloperidol, but otherwise very similar.
5. Indolones: molindone (Moban) is reported to have a lower incidence of extrapyramidal side effects.
6. Long-acting drugs: fluphenazine and haloperidol are available in decanoate form, which can be given at intervals of once a week to once a month.

III. ANTIDEPRESSANT DRUGS

The antidepressant drugs represent a class of medications that have the specific effect of elevating mood. They correct the biochemical imbalances that have been shown to exist in depressed individuals. in spite of this mood-elevating effect, antidepressants have little or no influence on the mood of a normal person. Since depression is one of

Table 20–1. ANTIPSYCHOTIC DRUGS

Drug Name	Dose Range
Chlorpromazine (Thorazine)	50–1000 mg/day
Thioridazine (Mellaril)	50–800 mg/day
Fluphenazine (Prolixin)	5–40 mg/day
Fluphenazine decanoate (Prolixin D)	25–100 mg IM Q1–3 weeks
Perphenazine (Trilafon)	4–64 mg/day
Trifluoperazine (Stelazine)	5–40 mg/day
Haloperidol (Haldol)	5–100 mg/day
Haloperidol decanoate (Haldol D)	50–200 mg IM Q2–4 weeks
Thiothixene (Navane)	5–60 mg/day
Loxapine (Loxitane)	20–250 mg/day
Molindone (Moban)	20–225 mg/day

the most commoly encountered psychiatric disorders, this group of psychotropic drugs is commonly used and highly effective.

Antidepressant agents can be loosely grouped into four categories: tricyclic antidepressants, tetracyclic antidepressants, monoamine oxidase inhibitors, and a group of new drugs that share various characteristics with the tricyclics.

A. Mechanism of Action

1. All of the antidepressant agents act, in one way or another, on the biogenic amines, norepinephrine and serotonin.
2. Early studies of depression found that the drug reserpine reduced the levels of serotonin and norepinephrine in the brain. This agent was also found to produce a clinical depression in many individuals.
3. Further studies of depressed patients have demonstrated reduced levels of biogenic amine metabolites in the urine of these individuals, implying a major role for these substances.
4. Tricyclic, tetracyclic, and the new antidepressants act by blocking the presynaptic reuptake of the biogenic amines, thus preventing their inactivation.
5. The monoamine oxidase inhibitors act to block the enzymatic degradation of the biogenic amines by the enzyme monoamine oxidase.

B. Indications

1. The antidepressants are effective in the treatment of a wide range of depressive disorders, ranging from the milder forms of depression to those accompanied by psychotic symptoms.
2. In addition to depression, some of the antidepressants (e.g., imipramine) have been found to be effective in the treatment of panic attacks and post-traumatic stress disorder.
3. Some evidence exists for the effectiveness of amitriptyline (and theoretically other antidepressants) in the treatment of chronic pain.

C. Side Effects and Toxicity

1. Antidepressants are contraindicated during the immediate post-myocardial infarction period because of their quinidine-like effect on the heart and the possibility of arrhythmias (see entry 7 below).
2. Tricyclic antidepressants and monoamine oxidase (MAO) inhibitors should be used in combination with great caution, because of reports of hypertensive crisis and sudden death.

3. Tricyclic and tetracyclic antidepressants both cause anticholinergic side effects similar to those seen with the antipsychotics.
4. Most of the antidepressants produce varying degrees of sedation.
5. The MAO inhibitors, and to a lesser extent the other antidepressants, may produce feelings of restlessness and agitation. Patients in the depressed phase of bipolar disorder may be thrown into a manic episode.
6. Antidepressants may precipitate a psychotic episode in susceptible individuals.
7. The tricyclic antidepressants are direct myocardial depressants and have quinidine-like effects. These cardiac effects include: prolonged conduction time, tachycardia, flattened T-waves, prolonged QT intervals, and depressed ST segments.

   At high doses or toxic levels, the tricyclics become arrhythmogenic. These drugs should be used with caution in patients with a history of cardiovascular disease.
8. Abrupt withdrawal from tricyclic antidepressants may cause temporary sleep disturbances.
9. The MAO inhibitors may cause a hypertensive crisis, which is often precipitated by eating foods containing high levels of tyramine. Individuals taking MAO inhibitors should avoid foods containing tyramine, as well as certain over-the-counter antihistamines and decongestants. Foods high in tyramine include beer and wine, aged cheeses, beef or chicken liver, smoked fish and herring, sausage, and fava or broad bean pods.

D. Specific Agents (see Table 20–2 for dose ranges)

1. Tricyclic antidepressants
   a. Amitriptyline (Elavil) is very sedating and has strong anticholinergic properties
   b. Imipramine (Tofranil) is less sedating but with prominent anticholinergic effects

Table 20–2. ANTIDEPRESSANT DRUGS

Drug Name	Dose Range
Amitriptyline (Elavil)	75–300 mg/day
Imipramine (Tofranil)	75–300 mg/day
Desipramine (Norpramin)	75–300 mg/day
Nortriptyline (Pamelor)	30–100 mg/day
Protriptyline (Vivactil)	15–40 mg/day
Doxepin (Sinequan)	50–300 mg/day
Maprotiline (Ludiomil)	75–150 mg/day
Amoxapine (Asendin)	50–300 mg/day
Trazodone (Desyrel)	100–400 mg/day
Tranylcypromine (Parnate)	20–60 mg/day
Phenelzine (Nardil)	60–90 mg/day

   c. Desipramine (Norpramin) has the fewest anticholinergic side effects of the tricyclics which often make them the drug of choice for elderly or debilitated patients
   d. Nortriptyline (Pamelor)
   e. Protriptyline (Vivactil)
   f. Doxepin (Sinequan) is also reported to have antianxiety effects
2. Tetracyclics: The only tetracyclic antidepressant currently in use is maprotiline (Ludiomil). This drug is reported to have fewer anticholinergic effects and to be less cardiotoxic than the tricyclics. It has been reported, however, to cause seizures at high doses.
3. MAO inhibitors
   a. Phenelzine (Nardil)
   b. Tranylcypromine (Parnate)
4. New antidepressants
   a. Amoxapine (Asendin) is a metabolite of the antipsychotic drug loxapine; as such it may have some antipsychotic activity. It may also cause extrapyramidal side effects. It is claimed to have a more rapid onset of action than other antidepressants.
   b. Trazodone (Desyrel) has fewer anticholinergic side effects and may be less cardiotoxic than the tricyclics. A rare side effect of trazodone in males is priapism.

IV. LITHIUM

Lithium is a psychotropic medication with a very specific action as a mood-stabilizing drug, and is the treatment of choice for the manic phase of bipolar disorder. It is unique among the various psychotropic medications because it lacks many of the bothersome side effects of the antipsychotics and antidepressants. Specifically, it has no sedative effect, does not cause troublesome anticholinergic effects, and does not lead to the development of tardive dyskinesia. As a result, lithium is better tolerated by most patients.

Lithium is also a drug that has been implicated in the treatment of several other psychiatric conditions. It has been the object of intense interest and study, although its effectiveness in other conditions remains unclear.

A. Mechanism of Action

1. The exact mechanism of action of lithium is unclear. It is thought to exert a stabilizing effect on central nervous system

neurons. This is most likely accomplished by stabilizing neuronal membranes.

2. As a result of this membrane stabilization, the release of norepinephrine is blocked and its reuptake is stimulated.

B. Indications

1. Lithium is the treatment of choice for the manic phase of bipolar disorders.
2. Lithium has also been shown to be effective preventing the cycles of depression associated with bipolar disorders.
3. Many patients with schizoaffective disorders, and some schizophrenics unresponsive to antipsychotics alone, improve when placed on lithium.
4. Some literature suggests that patients with various impulse-control disorders may benefit from lithium therapy.
5. There have been sporadic reports that lithium may be effective in the treatment of both alcoholism and borderline personality disorder. Conclusive evidence of this, however, is lacking.

C. Side Effects and Toxicity

1. Lithium has a clearly defined therapeutic range that can be measured in the serum. Therapeutic serum levels range from .05 to 1.5 mEq per liter. At levels above 1.5, toxic symptoms occur in most patients. These include: nausea and vomiting; abdominal cramps; diarrhea; polyuria and polydipsia, all at levels of 1.5 to 2; lethargy; coarse tremor and muscle twitching; ataxia; slurred speech; confusion; and convulsions, all at levels exceeding 2.0.
2. Renal damage may be associated with long-term lithium treatment. Nephrotoxicity usually affects tubular function, although glomerular function may rarely be impaired.
3. Lithium has several cardiac effects, including: T-wave flattening or inversion, similar to that seen with hypokalemia; arrhythmias; and congestive heart failure.

   A baseline ECG should always be obtained prior to initiating lithium therapy.
4. Mild hyperthyroidism, benign exophthalmus, and goiter occur in about 5% of patients taking lithium. Thyroid-stimulating hormone (TSH) levels may be elevated in these individuals.
5. Dermatological manifestations include an acneiform rash and a worsening of psoriasis.
6. Patients taking diuretics along with lithium may require a reduction in lithium dose, since diuretics cause an increase in lithium reabsorption.

D. Specific Agents

1. Lithium carbonate is administered in divided doses in a range of 900–2100 mg/day, monitoring serum levels.
2. Lithobid is a slow-release preparation that can be given twice a day instead of the usual three to four times a day.

V. ANTIANXIETY DRUGS AND SEDATIVE–HYPNOTICS

This group of drugs has strong antianxiety effects as well as producing sedation and sleep. A tremendous overlap exists between these agents, with the distinction between the antianxiety agents and the sedative-hypnotics often being quite arbitrary. In point of fact, these agents may often be used interchangeably, with dosage determining the desired effect.

Anxiety is a ubiquitous emotional experience. It becomes pathological only when it interferes with functioning. As such, most episodes of anxiety do not require treatment with medication. Antianxiety agents should only be used when the anxiety reaches a disabling proportion. Likewise, most sleep disturbances are transient and self-limiting. Use of these drugs to induce sleep should be a time-limited intervention.

A. Mechanism of Action

1. The benzodiazepines are the prototype for the antianxiety and sedative-hypnotic drugs. Much of our understanding of the biochemistry of anxiety has come from study of these drugs.
2. The benzodiazepines facilitate the synaptic actions of γ-aminobutyric acid (GABA), an inhibitory neurotransmitter. GABA apparently inhibits the firing of certain neurons, thereby decreasing anxiety. By augmenting the effect of GABA, the benzodiazepines reduce anxiety.
3. Further evidence in support of the hypothesis presented above comes from the discovery of specific benzodiazepine receptors in the brain, which exist in close proximity to GABA receptor sites.

B. Indications

1. Moderate to severe anxiety, from any source, is the primary indication for this group of drugs. It should be remembered, however, that anxiety is a normal affective experience. The presence of mild anxiety is not necessarily an indication for antianxiety medication.
2. Detoxification from alcohol is an important indication for the use of antianxiety drugs. The benzodiazepines are cross-tolerant

with alcohol. Chlordiazepoxide (Librium) has been the drug of choice; however, some treatment centers are now using the shorter-acting benzodiazepines.

3. Use of sedative-hypnotic drugs is indicated in the presence of moderate-to-severe sleep disturbances. As mentioned earlier, these drugs should be used for short-term treatment only.

C. Side Effects and Toxicity

1. The antianxiety and sedative-hypnotic drugs share similar side effect profiles.
2. As a group, these drugs are remarkably safe and free of side effects.
3. All members of this group have the potential for addiction and abuse. Long-term therapy at relatively high doses is needed before addiction to the benzodiazepines becomes a problem. Those drugs with longer half-lives present a greater risk for tolerance and addiction. The barbiturates, used primarily as sedative-hypnotic agents, have a greater potential for abuse and addiction than the benzodiazepines.
4. Because of the potential for habituation, these drugs should not be abruptly stopped. A gradual tapering of dose is recommended in order to prevent or decrease the severity of withdrawal symptoms.
5. Oversedation is a common side effect and is an indication for dose reduction.
6. Paradoxical agitation or excitement is a rarely seen side effect. Concurrent alcohol intake increases the likelihood of this reaction.
7. Abrupt withdrawal from barbiturates or from high-dose benzodiazepine therapy may precipitate grand mal seizures.

D. Specific Agents (see Table 20–3 for dose ranges)

1. Antianxiety agents: only the benzodiazepines will be considered. Drugs are listed in order of decreasing half-life:
   a. Diazepam (Valium)
   b. Chlordiazepoxide (Librium), the drug of choice for alcohol detoxification
   c. Clorazepate (Tranxene)
   d. Prazepam (Centrax)
   e. Halazepam (Paxipam)
   f. Lorazepam (Ativan)
   g. Alprazolam (Xanax), also has significant antidepressant action
   h. Oxazepam (Serax)

Table 20–3. ANTIANXIETY AND SEDATIVE–HYPNOTIC DRUGS

Drug Name	Dose Range
Antianxiety Drugs	
Diazepam (Valium)	4–40 mg/day
Chlordiazepoxide (Librium)	15–100 mg/day
Clorazepate (Tranxene)	15–16 mg/day
Prazepam (Centrax)	20–60 mg/day
Halazepam (Paxipam)	60–120 mg/day
Lorazepam (Ativan)	2–6 mg/day
Alprazolam (Xanax)	0.5–3.0 mg/day
Oxazepam (Serax)	30–120 mg/day
Sedative-Hypnotic Drugs	
Flurazepam (Dalmane)	15–30 mg/day
Chloral hydrate (Noctec)	500–1000 mg/day
Temazepam (Restoril)	15–30 mg/day
Secobarbital (Seconal)	100–200 mg/day
Triazolam (Halcion)	0.25–0.5 mg/day

2. Sedative-hypnotic agents
   a. Flurazepam (Dalmane), a benzodiazepine with very long half-life
   b. Chloral Hydrate (Noctec), a non-benzodiazepine, non-barbiturate sedative-hypnotic
   c. Temazepam (Restoril), a benzodiazepine
   d. Secobarbital (Seconal), a short-acting barbiturate
   e. Triazolam (Halcion), shortest-acting of the benzodiazepines

VI. SUMMARY

Five major classes of psychotropic medications exist, each with relatively specific effects on psychiatric symptoms: antipsychotic drugs, antidepressant drugs, lithium, antianxiety drugs, and sedative-hypnotics. Each class of drugs exerts direct effects on the central nervous system to modify behavior, mood, thought, and perception. Although many of these drugs have potentially serious side effects, when used in therapeutic doses they can effect a dramatic reversal of symptoms.

Although these medications are very effective, most patients require a combination of medication and some form of psychotherapy for optimal response. Timely interventions directed at the psychosocial aspects of psychiatric disorders significantly augment the effects of these medications.

References

Baldessarini, R. J. (1977). *Chemotherapy in psychiatry*. Cambridge: Harvard University Press.

Barklage, N. E., and Jefferson, J. W. (1987). Alternative uses of lithium in psychiatry. *Psychosomatics, 28,* 239–256.

Davis, J. M., and Maas, J. W. (1983). *The affective disorders.* Washington, DC: American Psychiatric Press.

Goodman, L. S., and Gilman, A. (Eds.). (1980). *The pharmacological basis of therapeutics* (6th ed.). New York: MacMillan.

Harris, E. (1981). Antipsychotic medications. *American Journal of Nursing, 81*(7), 1316–1323.

Harris, E. (1981). Extrapyramidal side effects. *American Journal of Nursing, 81*(7), 1324–1328.

Harris, E. (1981). Sedative-hypnotic drugs. *American Journal of Nursing, 81*(7), 1329–1334.

Jefferson, J. W., Griest, J. H., and Ackerman D. L. (1983). *Lithium encyclopedia for clinical practice.* Washington, DC: American Psychiatric Press.

Kaplan, H. I., and Sadock, B. J. (1985). *Comprehensive textbook of psychiatry* (4th ed.). New York: Williams & Wilkins.

Schultz, J. M., and Dark, S. L. (1986). *Manual of psychiatric nursing care plans* (2nd ed.). Boston: Little, Brown and Company.

Weinstein, M. R. (1978). Progress and problems: Antipsychotic, antidepressant and antianxiety drugs. *Hospital Formulary, 13,* 118–119.

Chapter 21

Legal Issues in Psychiatry

Theodore B. Feldmann

I. STATEMENT OF PURPOSE

This chapter is designed to give the nurse a basic introduction to legal issues in psychiatry. In recent years the legal system has had an increasing impact on all health care providers, with mental health professionals being no exception. Malpractice suits are at an all-time high. Physicians and hospitals are no longer the only target of these suits. All health care providers are now finding themselves the target of litigation, and professional liability insurance is now essential regardless of discipline. Health care providers are also being held accountable, to an increasing extent, for the actions of their patients. For example, therapists are now required to warn others of dangerous threats made by their patients. This development has radically altered the concept of confidentiality.

A brief overview of legal issues in psychiatry will be presented, followed by a review of landmark decisions that have had an impact on psychiatric care. Following this, a review of basic concepts and definitions will be presented. This material is intended as an introduction only. Specific laws vary from state to state. For information on the laws in your state, contact your state or local nursing association. In order to provide the necessary information, this chapter will follow an abbreviated format.

II. OVERVIEW

Over the years, psychiatrists have been involved in a number of legal issues, including those related to involuntary commitment, competency to manage one's personal affairs, criminal responsibility, competency to stand trial, and the right to compensation for psychological trauma or suffering. Recently, new issues related to dangerousness, duty to warn others, and the right to refuse treatment have surfaced. Questions of confidentiality are less clear-cut than in the past. As mentioned earlier, the threat of malpractice litigation is a concern of all professionals. This section will review some of the landmark decisions that have affected psychiatry in order to provide some background for the current issues surrounding mental health care.

A. M'Naghten Rule

One of the earliest decisions to influence psychiatry was the *M'Naghten Rule,* based on an 1843 English case. This decision became the standard for determining criminal responsibility and was adopted by many states. This rule states that in order to be found not guilty by reason of insanity, an individual must be found incapable of realizing the nature or severity of his act or of understanding that the act was wrong. The M'Naghten Rule was eventually abandoned and replaced by a new standard developed by the American Law Institute. The ALI test states, "It shall be a defense that the defendant at the time of the proscribed conduct, as a result of mental disease or defect, lacked substantial capacity either to appreciate the wrongfulness of his conduct or to conform his conduct to the requirements of the law."

B. Packard v. Illinois

The rights of involuntarily committed patients were expanded as the result of an 1860 Illinois case in which Elizabeth Packard was involuntarily hospitalized on the petition of her husband, without evidence of any mental illness. As a result of this abuse, states began mandating that patients receive due process before being committed.

C. Addington v. Texas

In the case of *Addington v. Texas* in 1979, the Supreme Court ruled that "clear and convincing" evidence must be presented before involuntary commitment could be ordered.

D. Lake v. Cameron

A 1966 decision in the case of *Lake v. Cameron* put forth the idea that committing courts must refrain from ordering hospitalization whenever a less restricting alternative exists. The concept of a "least restrictive alternative" has now been adopted by many states.

E. Rogers v. Comm. of Mental Health

The right to refuse treatment was upheld by the Massachusetts Supreme Court in the 1983 case of *Rogers v. Comm. of Mental Health.* This case specifically dealt with the right of a patient to refuse antipsychotic medication.

F. Dusky v. United States

The standards for determining competency to stand trial were set in the 1960 case of *Dusky v. United States.* This decision stated that in order to be determined competent to stand trial, an individual must understand the nature of the proceedings against him and be able to assist an attorney in the preparation of his defense.

G. Carter v. General Motors

The case of *Carter v. General Motors* allowed that individuals are entitled to compensation if stress or psychological trauma caused or exacerbated a psychiatric condition. In this particular case it was argued that the stress of working on an assembly line exacerbated a schizophrenic illness.

H. Wyatt v. Stickney

Wyatt v. Stickney, in 1972, focused attention on the substandard conditions in many state mental hospitals. This decision mandated that patients have a *right to treatment* if they are institutionalized. It determined that custodial care alone was not acceptable.

I. O'Connor v. Donaldson

The 1975 case of *O'Connor v. Donaldson* determined that mentally ill patients cannot be held involuntarily and without treatment if they are able to survive in society and are not dangerous.

J. Tarasoff Decision

The *Tarasoff decision* in California in 1976 mandated that therapists have the duty to warn individuals who are threatened by patients and have the duty to "exercise reasonable care to protect the forseeable victim of that danger."

These and many other similar decisions have placed greater burdens and responsibilities on mental health professionals to safeguard the rights of patients and others.

III. NURSING MANAGEMENT

An examination of legal issues in psychiatry introduces a variety of new and confusing terms. One of the great difficulties in dealing with legal issues involves mastering this new terminology. In order for nurses to deal with these issues effectively, however, the understanding of certain definitions is necessary. This section defines basic legal concepts that are frequently encountered in psychiatry. Guidelines for managing these issues are then presented.

A. Basic Concepts

1. *Tort* is the traditional legal term used to describe the commission of a wrongful act. The principle of tort forms the basis for malpractice claims. From a legal standpoint, tort represents a wrongful act that may entitle the victim to some type of compensation.
2. *Malpractice* refers to treatment that departs significantly from accepted, proper medical practice. This treatment results in either physical or psychological harm to the patient
3. The concept of *informed consent* states that treatment shall not be initiated, except under emergency conditions, without the full knowledge and consent of the patient. All risks and side effects need to be fully explained, and the patient needs to be advised of all alternative treatment methods. The idea of informed consent is closely linked to the right to refuse treatment.
4. Traditionally, physicians have been bound by the concept of *confidentiality,* which states that the physician must not disclose any information given by the patient. Psychotherapists have also considered information disclosed by the patient in therapy to be confidential. The courts, however, have been reluctant in many cases to grant the privilege of confidentiality to other health care providers. Recently, the courts have even begun to reconsider the concept of confidentiality as it applies to physicians. Successful suits have been brought against health care providers both for violating confidentiality and for failing to provide information. The latter instance applies especially where dangerousness is concerned (see entry 9 below).
5. *Competency* relates to an individual's ability to make sound decisions and to utilize good judgment. It is important to remember that the presence of a psychiatric disorder is not sufficient grounds for finding an individual incompetent. The determination of competency may relate to several areas, including the ability to manage one's own affairs and the ability to make decisions regarding consent to medical treatment.

6. *Abandonment* refers to the premature termination of treatment when further treatment would be beneficial and the failure to make provision for the patient to receive adequate treatment elsewhere.
7. *Involuntary commitment* refers to psychiatric hospitalization of an individual against his will. Specific criteria exist that must be met before a patient may be held against his will. These criteria are similar for all states. In general, an individual must be shown to suffer from a mental disorder of sufficient severity such that he represents a significant threat to self or others, or that his mental disorder prevents him from caring for himself and meeting his daily needs.
8. Although an individual may be hospitalized against his will, invasive treatments, such as forced IM medication, cannot be given without the consent of the patient. Likewise, a patient may not be restrained unless failure to do so would put the patient or others at risk for harm. From a legal standpoint, patients must be treated in the *least restrictive environment.*
9. Evaluation of *dangerousness* is a difficult and controversial area in mental health. The clinician's ability to predict violence is limited and is best related to a past history of violence. When an individual is determined to be dangerous, it is the responsibility of the health care provider to take sufficient steps to safeguard the patient and others. If specific threats are made, the professional must notify the intended victim and the authorities.

B. Nursing Planning and Intervention

1. The single most important element in dealing with legal issues is careful *documentation.* A complete and accurate medical record not only safeguards the nurse from legal issues but also improves patient care.
2. Notes should be clearly written, up-to-date, and objective. Report only clinical observations and concise descriptions of procedures. Avoid the use of emotional or derogatory statements.
3. Remember that many people have access to the patient's records. Therefore, use discretion in reporting sensitive material in the chart.
4. All forms of treatment must be clearly and carefully explained to the patient. Appropriate consent forms must be signed where required. Document in the chart that the treatment was discussed with the patient. When in doubt about a patient's understanding, have another staff member assist with the explanation.

5. When dealing with disturbed or agitated behavior, be sure to use the least restrictive means to assure the safety of both the patient and the staff. Seclusion and restraint should be used judiciously. Medication should not be forced unless the patient's behavior represents a clear threat to himself and others.
6. The best way to avoid complaints of malpractice or improper care is to maintain a sensitive and therapeutic relationship with the patient. Take time to listen to the patient's concerns and questions. Respect the patient's wishes and feelings.
7. The medical-surgical nurse should never *assume* that legal aspects of care have been attended to by another member of the health care team. Each nurse should have a working knowledge of the laws that pertain to her practice. Documentaion should specifically support any nursing interventions used for safety of the patient and others. Because a patient's chart is a legal document, reporting should be thorough and accurate.

IV. SUMMARY

Legal issues have become a concern to all health care providers. The practice of medicine and nursing have been radically altered by many recent court decisions. Claims awarded in malpractice settlements have reached staggering proportions. Awareness and understanding of legal issues is essential for all practitioners.

Providing adequate care, careful documentation, and common sense respect for the patient as an individual are the best ways of avoiding unnecessary legal difficulties.

References

Halleck, S. L. (1980). *Law in the practice of psychiatry*. New York: Plenum.

Kaplan, H. I., and Sadock, B. J. (1985). *Comprehensive textbook of psychiatry* 4th ed.). Baltimore: Williams & Wilkins.

Schultz, J. M., and Dark, S. L. (1986). *Manual of psychiatric nursing care plans* (2nd ed.). Boston: Little, Brown and Company.

Slovenko, R. (1973). *Psychiatry and law*. Boston: Little, Brown and Company.

Stuart, G. W. and Sunden, S. J. (1983). *Principles and practices of psychiatric nursing* (2nd ed.). St. Louis: C. V. Mosby Company.

Taylor, C. M. (1986). *Mereness' essentials of psychiatric nursing* (12th ed.). St. Louis: C. V. Mosby Company.

Appendix A

Psychosocial History

I. Identifying Data—name, age, race, marital status, occupation, referral source

II. Chief Complaint or Presenting Problem—informant, problem, onset, duration

III. History of the Present Problem—past and present psychiatric history, psychiatric admissions, psychiatric medications, family history of mental illness

IV. Past and Family History—developmental history, family background, siblings, marriages, children, education

V. Medical History—current medical problems, past history of accidents and surgeries, current medications, alcohol and drug use, family history of alcohol and drug use

VI. Military History—service dates, branch of service, areas stationed during service, drafted or volunteered, highest rank achieved, duties, any wounds or injuries, combat experience, any problems or disciplinary actions, type of discharge, service connected conditions, special commendations (see also Chapter 5, "The Patient with Post-Traumatic Stress Disorder")

VII. Legal History—current charges, past history of legal charges and/or imprisonment, problems or legal charges during youth and childhood

VIII. Present Life Status—employment, finances, residence

This suggested history is adapted from the patient history format developed by the staff of the Mental Hygiene Clinic at the Veterans Administration Medical Center in Huntington, West Virginia.

IX. Mental Status Examination (MSE)—See Appendix B, "Mental Status Examination"

X. Clinical Impression

XI. Nursing Diagnosis

XII. Recommendations and Treatment Plan

Appendix B

Mental Status Examination

The Mental Status Examination (MSE) is a way of assessing the patient's emotional and mental functioning.

I. **Appearance**—include manner of dress, grooming, general self-care, state of health, posture, facial expression, and any distinctive physical features (scars, tattoos, obesity or emaciation, and so on).

II. **Behavior**—degree of activity, cooperativeness, eye contact, distinct gestures or mannerisms, motor behavior, and general attitude. If the patient is on a psychotropic medication, look for extrapyramidal symptoms: tremor, grimacing, restlessness, pacing, foot tapping, hand-wringing, writhing or jerky movements of the tongue, mouth and jaw, trunk, and extremities.

III. **Speech**—rate of speech, tone, choice of words, lack of speech, degree of spontaneity, presence of abnormalities.

IV. **Thought**

A. **Content**—magical, bizarre, or unusual thought; delusional ideas of reference; grandiosity; paranoia; obsessions; preoccupation; suicidal or homicidal ideation.

B. **Process**—clarity of thought. Are thoughts logical and organized or are they tangential, circumstantial, or loosely associated (i.e, associations that are unrelated or disconnected)?

V. **Perceptions**—sensory awareness and interpretation of the environment; observe for illusions, hallucinations, depersonalization, and déjà vu.

VI. Mood and Affect

A. **Mood**—How does patient state that he feels (e.g., angry, depressed, elated, or anxious)?

B. **Affect**—What does the nurse observe about the patient's feelings—facial expression, demeanor, tone of voice, and body movement? Are mood and affect appropriate, constricted or blunted, flat, labile, and so on?

VII. Intellectual Functioning—A general impression can be formed from listening to the patient relate his history, but specific questions to assess intellectual function and memory should be asked.

A. **Orientation**—Time: year, season, date, and day of the week. Place: town, hospital, state, and country. Person: does the patient realize who he is? Can he give his name correctly?

B. **Registration and recall**—Can the patient recall the names of his nurse and physician? Name three to five unrelated objects and ask the patient to repeat them immediately and after 5 minutes (e.g., chair, the color blue, and New York City).

C. **Concentration**—Is the patient able to follow and carry out instructions? Ask the patient to perform serial 7's or 3's (i.e., what is 7 from 100; 7 from 93, and so on).

D. **Language**—Can the patient communicate verbally in a manner that is consistent with what the nurse knows the patient's educational background to be? Show the patient simple objects like a pen or watch and ask him to name them; have patient write a simple sentence.

E. **Long-term memory**—Have patient state his birthday, social security number, or other verifiable details of his life. Can the patient describe why he is in the hospital and what has happened to him?

F. **Thought processes**—Proverbs are often useful for detecting a subtle thought disorder. For example, ask patient to interpret the saying, "A rolling stone gathers no moss" or "People who live in glass houses shouldn't throw stones." Note concrete, bizarre, or nonsensical interpretations. Is the patient's train of thought logical and coherent or is it difficult to understand what he is trying to say?

G. **Insight**—Accurate assessment and understanding of his current situation. For example, a depressed patient who comes to the emergency room and is able to tell staff that he is depressed due to a specific loss or event and has insight into his situation.

H. **Judgment**—Ability to compare and assess alternatives, to make and carry out reasonable decisions, and to behave in an appropriate manner. A standard question in assessing judgment is "What would you do if you found an envelope that had a stamp and an address on it?" Most people would answer that they would put it in a mailbox. Answers that are inappropriate indicate impaired judgment.

Appendix C

DSM III-R Classification: Axes I and II Categories and Codes*

(See Axes Description at End)

Codes followed by an asterisk (*) are used for more than one DSM-III-R diagnosis or subtype. A long dash following a diagnostic term indicates the need for a fifth digit subtype or other qualifying term. NOS means "Not Otherwise Specified."

DISORDERS USUALLY FIRST EVIDENT IN INFANCY, CHILDHOOD, OR ADOLESCENCE

Developmental Disorders: (*Note*: These are coded on Axis II)

Mental Retardation

317.00 Mild mental retardation
318.00 Moderate mental retardation
318.10 Severe mental retardation
318.20 Profound mental retardation
319.00 Unspecified mental retardation

Pervasive Development Disorder

299.00 Autistic disorder
Specify if childhood onset
299.80 Pervasive developmental disorder NOS

*Reprinted with permission from the American Psychiatric Association (1987). Diagnostic and statistical manual of mental disorders *(3rd ed.—rev.). Washington, DC: American Psychiatric Association.*

Specific Developmental Disorders

Academic Skills Disorders

315.10 Developmental arithmetic disorder
315.80 Developmental expressive writing disorder
315.00 Developmental reading disorder

Language and Speech Disorders

315.39 Developmental articulation disorder
315.31* Developmental expressive language disorder
315.31* Developmental receptive language disorder

Motor Skills Disorder

315.40 Developmental coordination disorder
315.90* Specific developmental disorder NOS

Other Developmental Disorders

315.90* Developmental disorder NOS

Disruptive Behavior Disorders

314.01 Attention-deficit hyperactivity disorder
Conduct disorder,
312.20 group type
312.00 solitary aggressive type
312.90 undifferentiated type
313.81 Oppositional defiant disorder

Anxiety Disorders of Childhood or Adolescence

309.21 Separation anxiety disorder
313.21 Avoidant disorder of childhood or adolescence
313.00 Overanxious disorder

Eating Disorders

307.10 Anorexia nervosa
307.51 Bulimia nervosa
307.52 Pica
307.53 Rumination disorder of infancy
307.50 Eating disorder NOS

Gender Identity Disorders

302.60 Gender identity disorder of childhood
302.50 Transsexualism
Specify sexual history, asexual, homosexual, heterosexual, unspecified
302.85* Gender identity disorder of adolescence or childhood, nontranssexual type
Specify sexual history, asexual, homosexual, heterosexual, unspecified
302.85* Gender identity disorder NOS

Tic Disorders

307.23 Tourette's disorder
307.22 Chronic motor or vocal tic disorder
307.21 Transient tic disorder
Specify: single episode or recurrent
307.20 Tic disorder NOS

Elimination Disorders

307.7 Functional encopresis
Specify: primary or secondary type
307.60 Functional enuresis
Specify: primary or secondary type
Specify: nocturnal only, diurnal only, nocturnal and diurnal

Speech Disorders Not Elsewhere Classified

307.00* Cluttering
307.00* Stuttering

Other Disorders of Infancy, Childhood, or Adolescence

313.20 Elective mutism
313.82 Identity disorder
313.89 Reactive attachment disorder of infancy or early childhood
307.30 Stereotypy/habit disorder
314.00 Undifferentiated attention deficit disorder

ORGANIC MENTAL DISORDERS

Dementias Arising in the Senium and Presenium

Primary degenerative dementia or the Alzheimer type, senile onset,
290.30 with delirium
290.20 with delusions
290.21 with depression
290.00 uncomplicated
(*Note:* code 331.00 Alzheimer's dsease on Axis III)

Code in fifth digit: 1 = with delirium, 2 = with delusions, 3 = with depression, 0* = uncomplicated

290.1x Primary degenerative dementia of the Alzheimer type, presenile onset, ______
(*Note:* code 331.00 Alzheimer's disease on Axis III)
290.4x Multi-infarct dementia, ______
290.00* Senile dementia NOS
Specify etiology on Axis III if known (e.g., Pick's disease, Creutzfeld-Jakob disease)

Psychoative Substance–Induced Organic Mental Disorders

Alcohol
303.00 intoxication
291.40 idiosyncratic intoxication
291.80 Uncomplicated alcohol withdrawal
291.00 withdrawal delirium
291.20 hallucinosis
291.10 amnestic disorder
291.20 Dementia associated with alcoholism

Amphetamine or similarly acting sympathomimetic
305.70* intoxication
292.00* withdrawal
292.81* delirium
292.11* delusional disorder

Caffeine
305.90* intoxication

Cannabis
305.20* intoxication
292.11* delusional disorder

Cocaine
305.60* intoxication
292.00* withdrawal
292.81* delirium
292.11* Posthallucinogen perception disorder

Inhalant
305.90* intoxication

Nicotine
292.00* withdrawal

Opioid
305.50* intoxication
292.00* withdrawal

Phencyclidine (PCP) or similarly acting arylcyclohexylamine
305.90* intoxication
292.81* delirium
292.11* delusional disorder
292.84* mood disorder
292.90* organic mental disorder NOS

Sedative, hypnotic, or anxiolytic
305.40* intoxication
292.00* Uncomplicated sedative, hypnotic, or anxiolytic withdrawal

292.00* withdrawal delirium
292.83* amnestic disorder

Other or unspecified psychoactive substance
305.90* intoxication
292.00* withdrawal
292.81* delirium
292.82* dementia
292.83* amnestic disorder
292.11* delusional disorder
292.12* hallucinosis
292.84* mood disorder
292.89* anxiety disorder
292.89* personality disorder
292.90* organic mental disorder NOS

Organic Mental Disorder Associated with Axis III Physical Disorders or Conditions, or Whose Etiology Is Unknown

293.00 Delirium
294.10 Dementia
294.00 Amnestic disorder
293.81 Organic delusional disorder
392.82 Organic hallucinosis
293.83 Organic mood disorder
Specify: manic, depressed, mixed
294.80* Organic anxiety disorder
310.10 Organic personality disorder
294.80* Organic mental disorder NOS

PSYCHOACTIVE SUBSTANCE USE DISORDERS

Alcohol
303.90 dependence
205.00 abuse

Amphetamine or similarly acting sympathomimetic
304.40 dependence
305.70* abuse

Cannabis
304.30 dependence
305.20* abuse

Cocaine
304.20 dependence
305.60* abuse

Hallucinogen
304.50* dependence
305.30* abuse

Inhalant
304.60 dependence
305.90* abuse

Nicotine
205.10 dependence

Opioid
304.00 dependence
305.50* abuse

Phencyclidine (PCP) or similarly acting arylcyclohexylamine
304.50* dependence
305.90* abuse

Sedative, hypnotic, or anxiolytic
304.10 dependence
305.40* abuse
304.90* Polysubstance dependence
304.90* Psychoactive substance dependence NOS
305.90* Psychoactive substance abuse NOS

SCHIZOPHRENIA

Code in fifth digit: 1 = subchronic, 2 = chronic, 3 = subchronic with acute exacerbation, 4 = chronic with acute exacerbation, 5 = in remission, 0 = unspecified.

Schizophrenia,
295.2x catatonic, ______
295.1x disorganized, ______
295.3x paranoid, ______
Specify if stable type
295.9x undifferentiated, ______
295.6x residual, ______
Specify if late onset

DELUSIONAL (PARANOID) DISORDER

297.10 Delusional (Paranoid) disorder
Specify type: erotamanic
grandiose
jealous
persecutory
somatic
unspecified

PSYCHOTIC DISORDERS NOT ELSEWHERE CLASSIFIED

298.80 Brief reactive psychosis
295.40 Schizophreniform disorder
  Specify: without good prognostic features or with good prognostic features
295.70 Schizoaffective disorder
  Specify: bipolar type or depressive type
297.30 Induced psychotic disorder
298.90 Psychotic disorder NOS (Atypical psychosis)

MOOD DISORDERS

Code current state of Major Depression and Bipolar Disorder in fifth digit:

1 = mild
2 = moderate
3 = severe, without psychotic features
4 = with psychotic features (specify mood-congruent or mood-incongruent
5 = in partial remission
6 = in full remission
0 = unspecified

For major depressive episodes, specify if chronic and specify if melancholic type.
For Bipolar Disorder, Bipolar Disorder NOS, Recurrent Major Depression, and Depressive Disorder NOS, specify if seasonal pattern.

Bipolar Disorders

Bipolar disorder,
296.6x mixed, ______
296.4x manic, ______
296.5x depressed, ______
301.13 Cyclothymia
296.70 Bipolar disorder NOS

Depressive Disorders

Major depression,
296.2x single episode, ______
296.3x recurrent, ______
300.40 Dysthymia (or depressive neurosis)
  Specify: primary or secondary type
  Specify: early or late onset
311.00 Depressive disorder NOS

ANXIETY DISORDERS (or Anxiety and Phobic Neuroses)

Panic disorder
300.21 with agoraphobia

Specify current severity of agoraphobic avoidance
Specify current severity of panic attacks
300.01 without agoraphobia
Specify current severity of panic attacks
300.22 Agoraphobia with history of panic disorder
Specify with or without limited symptom attacks
300.23 Social phobia
Specify if generalized type
300.29 Simple phobia
300.30 Obsessive compulsive disorder (or Obsessive compulsive neurosis)
309.89 Post-traumatic stress disorder
Specify if delayed onset
300.02 Generalized anxiety disorder
300.00 Anxiety disorder

SOMATOFORM DISORDERS

300.70* Body dysmorphic disorder
300.11 Conversion disorder (or Hysterical neurosis, conversion type)
Specify: single episode or recurrent
300.70* Hypochondriasis (or Hypochondriacal neurosis)
300.81 Somatization disorder
307.80 Somatoform pain disorder
300.70* Undifferentiated somatoform disorder
300.70* Somatoform disorder NOS

DISSOCIATIVE DISORDERS (or Hysterical Neuroses, Dissociative Type)

300.14 Multiple personality disorder
300.13 Psychogenic fugue
300.12 Psychogenic amnesia
300.60 Depersonalization disorder (or Depersonalization neurosis)
300.15 Dissociative disorder NOS

SEXUAL DISORDERS

Paraphilias
302.40 Exhibitionism
302.81 Fetishism
302.89 Frotteurism
302.20 Pedophilia
Specify: same sex, opposite sex, same and opposite sex
Specify if limited to incest
Specify: exclusive type or nonexclusive type
302.83 Sexual masochism

302.84 Sexual sadism
302.30 Transvestic fetishism
302.82 Voyeurism
302.90* Paraphilia NOS

Sexual Dysfunctions

Specify: psychogenic only, or psychogenic and biogenic (*Note:* If biogenic only, code on Axis III)
Specify: lifelong or acquired
Specify: generalized or situational

Sexual desire disorders
302.71 Hypoactive sexual desire disorder
302.79 Sexual aversion disorder
Sexual arousal disorders
302.72* Female sexual arousal disorder
302.72* Male erectile disorder
Orgasm disorders
302.73 Inhibited female orgasm
302.74 Inhibited male orgasm
302.75 Premature ejaculation
Sexual pain disorders
302.76 Dyspareunia
306.51 Vaginismus
302.70 Sexual dysfunction NOS

Other Sexual Disorders

302.90* Sexual disorder NOS

SLEEP DISORDERS

Dyssomnias

Insomnia disorder
307.42* related to another mental disorder (nonorganic)
780.50* related to known organic factor
307.42* Primary insomnia
Hypersomnia disorder
307.44 related to another mental disorder (nonorganic)
780.50* related to known organic factor
780.54 Primary hypersomnia
307.45 Sleep-wake schedule disorder
Specify: advanced or delayed phase type, disorganized type, frequently changing type
Other dyssomnias
307.40* Dyssomnia NOS

Parasomnias

307.47 Dream anxiety disorder (nightmare disorder)
307.46* Sleep terror disorder

307.46* Sleepwalking disorder
307.40* Parasomnia NOS

FACTITIOUS DISORDERS

Factitious disorder
301.51 with physical symptoms
300.16 with psychological sypmtoms
300.19 Factitious disorder NOS

IMPULSE CONTROL DISORDERS NOT ELSEWHERE CLASSIFIED

312.34 Intermittent explosive disorder
312.32 Kleptomania
312.31 Pathological gambling
312.33 Pyromania
312.39* Trichotillomania
312.39* Impulse control disorder NOS

ADJUSTMENT DISORDER

Adjustment disorder
309.24 with anxious mood
309.00 with depressed mood
309.30 with disturbance of conduct
309.40 with mixed disturbance of emotions and conduct
309.28 with mixed emotional features
309.82 with physical complaints
309.83 with withdrawal
309.23 with work (or academic) inhibition
309.90 Adjustment disorder NOS

PSYCHOLOGICAL FACTORS AFFECTING PHYSICAL CONDITION

316.00 Psychological factors affecting physical condition
Specify physical condition on Axis III

PERSONALITY DISORDERS

Note: These are coded on Axis II.
Cluster A
301.00 Paranoid
301.20 Schizoid
301.22 Schizotypal

Cluster B
301.70 Antisocial
301.83 Borderline
301.50 Histrionic
301.81 Narcissistic
Cluster C
301.82 Avoidant
301.60 Dependent
301.40 Obsessive compulsive
301.84 Passive aggressive
301.90 Personality disorder NOS

V CODES FOR CONDITIONS NOT ATTRIBUTABLE TO A MENTAL DISORDER THAT ARE A FOCUS OF ATTENTION OR TREATMENT

V62.30 Academic problem
V71.01 Adult antisocial behavior
V40.00 Borderline intellectual functioning (*Note:* This is coded on Axis II.)
V71.02 Childhood or adolescent antisocial behavior
V65.20 Malingering
V61.10 Marital problem
V15.81 Noncompliance with medical treatment
V62.20 Occupational problem
V61.20 Parent-child problem
V62.81 Other interpersonal problem
V61.80 Other specified family circumstances
V62.89 Phase of life problem or other life circumstance problem
V62.82 Uncomplicated bereavement

ADDITIONAL CODES

300.90 Unspecified mental disorder (nonpsychotic)
V71.09* No diagnosis or condition on Axis I
799.90* Diagnosis or condition deferred on Axis I
V71.09* No diagnosis or condition on Axis II
799.90* Diagnosis or condition deferred on Axis II

MULTIAXIAL SYSTEM

Axis I Clinical Syndrome V Codes
Axis II Developmental Disorders
Personality Disorders
Axis III Physical Disorders and Conditions
Axis IV Severity of Psychosocial Stressors
Axis V Global Assessment of Functioning

Appendix D

Table of Psychoactive Drugs

Classification	Effects	Dangers	Withdrawal Symptoms	Treatment
Narcotics Heroin Morphine Methadone Opium Demerol Dilaudid Talwin Codeine	Drowsiness Respiratory depression Relaxation Euphoria Impaired judgment Low energy level Passivity Constipation Pinpoint pupils Nausea and vomiting Stupor	Addiction Loss of appetite with malnutrition Tolerance Mental deterioration Convulsions Respiratory failure Possible death Severe withdrawal symptoms Strong craving for the drug Hepatitis or AIDS from shared or dirty needles Intravascular infection	Similar to a "bad" case of the flu; major symptoms last 5–7 days or longer. Itching Irritability Anxiety Muscle twitching Tremors Sneezing Yawning Sweating Nausea and vomiting Fever Leg and abdominal cramps Dehydration Withdrawal from street drugs may be complicated by convulsions due to the poor quality of drugs and adulterants used to "cut" the drugs.	Gradual withdrawal of the drug being abused or methadone substitution and detoxification. Most detoxification can be accomplished in 7–10 days, with 21 days being the maximum allowed by the Food and Drug Administration (FDA). Propoxyphene (Darvon) is used by some to detoxify opiate addicts. Clonidine (Catapres) has been used with some success as an adjunct to control sympathetic overactivity resulting from opiate withdrawal.

Table continued on following page

Appendix D—Table of Psychoactive Drugs—*Continued*

Classification	Effects	Dangers	Withdrawal Symptoms	Treatment
Stimulant/Narcotic Cocaine	Excitation Increased alertness Sensation of pleasure Talkativeness Euphoria Anxiety Restlessness Extreme irritability Strong cravings Prolonged sleep Fatigue Depression Hunger	Addiction Tolerance Depression Psychological dependence Reverse tolerance Personality changes Tachycardia Hypertension Ventricular arrhythmias Respiratory failure Grand mal seizures Acute anxiety Psychosis Hallucinations Ideas of reference Paranoia Sexual dysfunction Compulsive sexual acting-out Death	Intense craving for the drug Depression Agitation Lethargy Insomnia Irritability Following a brief high-dose binge, a 2–4 hour period of: apathy, depression, fatigue, and exhaustion may be noted. Following chronic use of high doses: dysphoric mood, lethargy, insomnia, and irritability may be noted.	Treatment of acute cocaine overdose is specific to the symptoms, including seizures and cardiac arrhythmias. For anxiety with elevated pulse and blood pressure, diazepam or propranolol may be used. Severe depression may require use of tricyclic antidepressants. Allow sleep for extended periods. Provide a nutritious diet.

Stimulant Amphetamine Methamphetamine	Increased activity Exhilaration Decreased appetite Aggressive behavior Silliness Rapid speech Confusion Fatigue Anxiety Agitation Weight loss Tachycardia Dilated pupils Elevated blood pressure Tremulousness Sweating Fever Hyperreflexia Dry mouth Extreme restlessness and irritability	Addiction Tolerance Psychosis Paranoia Hallucinations Violence Psychological dependence May feel fearless and take risks Exhaustion Visual distortion Possible death	Lethargy Somnolence Depression with suicidal ideation	Quiet environment Decreased sensory stimulation Allow sleep Close observation Hospitalization and treatment with antipsychotics if necessary. Suicide precautions if necessary. Acidification of the urine may promote more rapid clearing of psychosis due to decreased half-life of the drug.

Table continued on following page

Appendix D—Table of Psychoactive Drugs—*Continued*

Classification	Effects	Dangers	Withdrawal Symptoms	Treatment
Sedatives/hypnotics Barbiturates Benzodiazepines Methaqualone etc.	Euphoria Intoxication Drowsiness Sleep Poor coordination Respiratory depression Hypotension Impaired judgment Decreased heart rate Staggering Slurred speech Tremors Irritability Dullness of mental processes	Addiction Depression with suicidal ideation Anxiety Loss of consciousness Coma Seizures Possible death Falling asleep while driving Slowed reflexes Intoxication Stupor Psychological dependence Severe withdrawal symptoms followed by a very slow recovery.	Withdrawal from sedative/hypnotics can be more ravaging than withdrawal from heroin. Agitation Anxiety Panic attacks Weakness Tachycardia Sweating Insomnia Muscle twitching Nausea and vomiting Diarrhea Hypotension Disorientation Confusion Hallucinations Delirium Grand mal seizures Death can occur from abrupt withdrawal.	Withdrawal should be done in a hospital under medical supervision with decreasing doses of the same or a similar drug. Careful observation for convulsions is crucial.

Hallucinogens Lysergic acid diethylamide (LSD) Phencyclidine (PCP) Dimethyltryptamine (DMT) Mescaline Psilocybin Marihuana in high doses	Altered perceptions Sensory distortion Distortion of reality Euphoria Confusion Grandiose feelings Relaxation Decreased inhibitions Exhilaration Bizarre behavior Feelings of detachment Slurred or incoherent speech Vomiting Chills Cold, sweaty hands and feet Irregular respirations Anxiety Delirium Paranoia Poor coordination Erratic emotions	Panic Flashbacks Psychosis Hallucinations Delusions Depression Paranoia Suicidal tendencies Tolerance develops quickly Chromosomal damage Prolonged psychotic reaction	Initially the patient may fall into a restless sleep. Watering of eyes and nose Yawning Sweating Gooseflesh Back and stomach cramps Nausea and vomiting Fever Diarrhea Twitching of leg muscles Symptoms are most pronounced during the first 72 hours and are flu-like. Flashbacks and prolonged psychosis may require ongoing treatment.	Management of adverse or toxic reactions. Give calm reassurance. Hospitalization if necessary. Medication should be used sparingly.

Table continued on following page

Appendix D—Table of Psychoactive Drugs—*Continued*

Classification	Effects	Dangers	Withdrawal Symptoms	Treatment
Deliriant* Glue Toluene Inhalants Fingernail polish remover Cleaning fluid Lighter fluid Paint thinner Aerosols Gasoline	Sensory distortion Hallucinations Depression Intoxicated appearance Staggering Slurred speech Double vision Buzzing in ears Headache Nausea and vomiting Violence Stupor Poor muscle coordination Dreamy or blank expression Excess nasal secretions Tearing of eyes Sedation of CNS	Seizures Damage to brain, liver, kidneys, bone marrow, and lungs Can go from drowsiness to coma Amnesia Suffocation Death	Rebound excitement (even to the point of delirium) Tremors Anxiety Restlessness (The nurse will need to question the patient for these symptoms, as he may not volunteer this information.)	Possible use of an oral sedative drug like one of the benzodiazepines for gradual withdrawal. For choking and/or suffocation, use supportive measures to maintain patent airway/respiration.

*Symptoms are based on clinical observation and pharmacological properties of deliriants. Although there are no clinical reports, theoretically speaking, the nurse might expect a full-blown withdrawal syndrome like that seen in delirium tremens.

Euphoriant Marihuana	Talkative Hilarious mood Enlarged pupils Poor coordination Increased appetite Craving for sweets Erratic behavior Memory lapses Distortion of time and space Relaxation Euphoria Decreased inhibitions Hallucinations Slowed reaction time Impaired judgment	Behaving in a manner dangerous to self or others Accident proneness Damage to brain, reproductive organs, lungs, and liver. Psychosis Hallucinations Probable psychological dependence Could lead to use of stronger drugs	Some experts have noted a withdrawal syndrome associated with use of marihuana. Adverse behavioral reactions may occur as panic attacks, psychosis, or organic brain syndrome. Panic attacks are generally associated with fear of losing control or going crazy. Psychosis may be associated with visual hallucinations and violence.	**Panic attacks:** close observation quiet room calm approach possible use of benzodiazepines such as chlordiazepoxide (Librium) **Psychosis:** Hospitalization; take appropriate precautions if dangerous to self or others; use of an antipsychotic such as haloperidol (Haldol).

*Glossary**

Abstract thinking—The ability to arrive at a conclusion from a logical reasoning process.

Acting-Out—The expression of unconscious feelings and fantasies in behavior. Often applied somewhat imprecisely to any sort of disapproved impulsive behavior.

Affect—An external expression of emotion attached to ideas or mental representation of objects. See *Mood.*

Aggression—A form of behavior that leads to self-assertion; it may be manifested by destructive and attacking behavior, by covert attitudes of hostility and obstructionism, or by a healthy self-expressive drive to mastery.

Agitation—A state of anxiety accompanied by motor restlessness.

Akathisia—A condition of motor restlessness in which there is a feeling of muscular quivering, an urge to move about constantly, and an inability to sit still. A feeling of intense inner restlessness. (A common side effect of antipsychotic drugs.)

Alloplastic—Adaptation by alteration of the external environment, i.e., the individual expects the external world to change and adapt to him.

Ambivalence—The simultaneous existence of conflicting attitudes, emotions, ideas, or wishes toward the same object.

Anorexia nervosa—A mental disorder occurring predominantly in females and characterized by a refusal to maintain a normal minimal body weight, an intense fear of obesity, a disturbance in body image, and amenorrhea (in females). Death from starvation may occur.

Antipsychotic—A class of drugs used to treat schizophrenic, paranoid, schizoaffective, and other psychotic disorders; acute delirium and dementia; and manic episodes. Also called neuroleptics and major tranquilizers.

Anxiety—An unpleasant emotional state consisting of psychophysiological responses to anticipation of real or imagined danger. Psychological reactions include increased heart rate, altered respiratory rate, sweating,

*Terms in the Glossary are based on *Dorland's Illustrated Medical Dictionary* (27th Ed.). Philadelphia: W. B. Saunders Co., (1988).

trembling, weakness, and fatigue. Psychological aspects include feelings of impending danger, powerlessness, fear, apprehension, and tension.

Anxiolytic—An agent that reduces anxiety.

Autogenic relaxation—Inducing relaxation in one's self through use of internal stimuli such as visual imagery and internal dialogue. Gradual, progressive relaxation of voluntary muscles, usually starting with the toes and feet and progressing upward to include the entire body.

Autoplastic—Adaptation by changing one's self; i.e., the individual attempts to adapt to the environment around him.

Behavior modification—A form of treatment in which undesired behavior patterns are changed to more desirable responses by a system of rewarding desired behavior and not rewarding undesired behavior.

Biofeedback—The process of furnishing information to an individual, usually visual or auditory, on the state of one or more physiological variables such as heart rate, blood pressure, or skin temperature. This procedure often enables the individual to gain some voluntary control over the variable being sampled. Often used to promote relaxation and as an adjunct to pain management.

Bipolar disorder—A mood disorder characterized by severe mood swings alternating between elated, manic episodes, and major depressive episodes. There is often a family history of bipolar disorder.

Buccofacialmandibular—Involving the tongue, face, and jaw.

Buccolingual—Pertaining to the cheek and tongue.

Bulimia—A mental disorder, occurring predominantly in females, characterized by episodes of binge eating that continue until terminated by abdominal pain, sleep, or self-induced vomiting. The individual is aware that the binges are abnormal, and binges may alternate with periods of normal eating or fasting.

Catatonic—A condition characterized by a fixed, immobile posture.

Choreoathetoid—A combination of the clinical features seen in both chorea and athetosis. This condition is marked by a wide variety of irregular, jerky movements and slow, writhing movements.

Circumstantiality—A pattern of speech characterized by delay in getting to the point because of the inclusion of unnecessary, tedious, and irrelevant details.

Concrete thinking—Interpreting what one sees and hears in a rigid, inflexible manner. Inability to use abstract thinking to determine meanings.

Confabulation—The "filling in" of gaps in one's memory by imaginary or fantastic experiences. These are recounted in a detailed and plausible manner as if they actually occurred.

Confusion—Disorientation to time, place, and/or person.

Countertransference—A transference reaction of therapist to patient; i.e., an emotional reaction that is a reflection of the therapist's own inner needs and conflicts. See *Transference*.

Cyclothymic—Describing a mood disorder characterized by numerous hypomanic and depressive periods with symptoms like those of manic and major depressive episodes but of lesser severity.

Decompensation—Failure of defense mechanisms, resulting in progressive personality disintegration.

Defense mechanisms—Automatic, generally unconscious measures taken to ensure self-protection against unwanted thoughts and feelings or reality.

Delirium—An acute, reversible organic mental disorder characterized by decreased ability to maintain attention to external stimuli and by disorganized thinking. Manifested by rambling; irrelevant or incoherent speech; reduced level of consciousness; sensory misperceptions; disturbance in sleep-wakefulness cycle and level of psychomotor activity; disorientation to time, place, and/or person; and memory impairment.

Delirium tremens—Caused by cessation or reduction in alcohol consumption. Clinical manifestations include autonomic hyperactivity, such as tachycardia, sweating, and hypertension; a coarse, irregular tremor; vivid hallucinations; and wild, agitated behavior. Also called alcohol withdrawal syndrome.

Delusion—A false belief that is firmly maintained in spite of obvious evidence to the contrary and in spite of the fact that other members of the culture do not share the belief.

Dementia—An organic mental disorder characterized by a general loss of intellectual abilities involving impairment of memory, judgment, and abstract thinking, as well as changes in personality.

Denial—A defense mechanism in which the existence of unpleasant realities is kept out of conscious awareness.

Depersonalization—Feeling strange or unreal.

Disequilibrium—A condition in which the checks and balances among the interdependent parts (family members) of a system become threatened and out of balance.

Dissociation—A defense mechanism in which a group of mental processes are segregated from the rest of a person's mental activity in order to avoid emotional distress.

Dysphoria—Disquiet, restlessness, malaise. Excessive pain, anguish, and agitation.

Dysphoric—Characterized by dysphoria.

Dysthymic disorder—A mood disorder characterized by depression and loss of interest or pleasure in one's usual activities and in which the associated symptoms have persisted for more than two years but are not severe enough to meet DSM III-R criteria for major depression.

Ego-dystonic or ego-alien—Aspects of a person's thoughts, impulses, attitudes, and behavior that are felt to be distressing, unacceptable, or inconsistent with the rest of his personality.

Ego-syntonic—Part of the ego. Aspects of a person's thoughts, impulses, attitudes, and behavior that are felt to be acceptable and consistent with the rest of his personality.

Electroconvulsive therapy (ECT)—Inducing convulsions by means of electric shock.

Elopement—A term that is used to describe a patient's leaving the hospital without permission and without having been discharged. Running away from the hospital.

Euphoria—An exaggerated and inappropriate feeling of physical and mental well-being.

Extrapyramidal symptoms (EPS)—Side effects of antipsychotic drugs that resemble symptoms of Parkinson's disease. May include tremor, drooling, and altered gait.

Flight of ideas—A nearly continuous flow of rapid speech that jumps from topic to topic.

Hallucination—A sense perception without a source in the external world. It may be auditory, visual, olfactory, tactile, or gustatory.

Homeostasis (family)—A balance process in which the family members keep each other in check, always returning the family system to its steady state.

Homicidal ideation—Thoughts of taking the life of another person.

Ideas of reference—The assumption by a patient that the words and actions of others refer specifically to himself. The patient may believe that a television or radio program or a newspaper article may be referring directly to him.

Illusion—A false intepretation of a real sensory image

Imagery—Mental visualization of persons, places, or objects.

Judgment—The ability of an individual to behave in a socially appropriate way.

Labile—Emotional instability; rapidly changing emotions.

Loose associations—A disorder of thinking in which ideas expressed are fragmented and are unrelated or only slightly related.

Major depression—A mental disorder characterized by the occurrence of one or more major depressive episodes and the absence of any history of manic episodes. Symptoms are severe enough to interfere with the individual's functioning and must have persisted for longer than two weeks. Symptoms include depressed mood; loss of interest or pleasure; weight change; sleep disturbance; fatigue; feelings of worthlessness or excessive guilt; difficulty with memory and concentration; psychomotor agitation or retardation; and recurrent thoughts of death.

Manic depressive disorder—See *Bipolar affective disorder.*

Mental status exam—A means of evaluating abnormalities in the level of consciousness, thinking, feeling, perception, memory, and behavior of the patient.

Mood—A pervasive and sustained emotion that, when extreme, can color one's entire view of life. When comparing mood and affect, mood can be thought of as climate, and affect as current weather conditions.

Neuroleptic—A term referring to the cognitive and behavioral effects of antipsychotic drugs, which produce a state of apathy, lack of initiative, and limited range of emotion and which in psychotic patients can cause a reduction in confusion and agitation, and normalization of psychomotor activity.

Neurosis—A mental disorder in which reality testing is intact and egodystonic symptoms, such as obsessions, anxiety attacks, phobias, and somatoform symptoms, occur.

Neurotransmitters—Any group of chemical substances that convey electrical impulses from one neuron to another. This group includes serotonin, norepinephrine, dopamine, and acetylocholine.

Noncompliance—Failure to cooperate with the therapeutic plan. The patient's behavior may be self-destructive.

Oculogyric crisis—A condition in which the eyeballs become fixed in one position for minutes or hours.

Opisthotonos—A form of spasm in which the head and the heels are bent backward and the body bowed forward.

Overfunctioning (family member)—An overly responsible family member who dominates the relationship in terms of decisions that effect the others in order to preserve a common self. See *Underfunctioning.*

Paranoia—A psychotic disorder marked by persistent delusions of persecution or delusional jealousy. Behavior such as suspiciousness, mistrust, and combativeness may be seen.

Parkinsonism—A group of neurological disorders characterized by hypokinesia, fine tremor, and muscular rigidity.

Passive-aggressive behavior—An immature defense mechanism in which a person's hostility and anger are expressed indirectly or covertly in ways that are often self-defeating and in some way offensive to the other.

Personality—The characteristic manner in which a person thinks, feels, and behaves. It is relatively stable and predictable. It includes conscious attitudes, values, and style as well as unconsious conflicts and defense mechanisms.

Personality disorder—Specific mental disorders composed of inflexible and maladaptive personality traits that are self-perpetuating, generate subjective distress, and result in significant impairments in social functioning.

Phobia—A persistent, irrational, and intense fear of a specific object, activity, or situation.

Pseudodementia—A disorder resembling dementia that is not due to organic brain disease and can be reversed with treatment.

Psychosis—A mental disorder characterized by gross impairment in reality testing.

Reaction formation—An unconscious defense mechanism in which an individual assumes an attitude that is the reverse of a wish or impulse that he harbors.

Reality testing—A basic ego function that consists of the objective evaluation and judgment of the world outside of the self.

Recent memory—The ability to recall events from the immediate past. It is generally affected first in memory loss.

Regression—A return to earlier, especially to infantile, patterns of thought or behavior.

Remote memory—The ability to recall events from the distant past.

Schizoaffective—Exhibiting features of both schizophrenic and mood disorders (mania and depression).

Schizophrenia—A severe thought disorder of psychotic depth characterized by a retreat from reality with the formation of delusions and hallucinations, emotional disharmony, regression, poor communication, and impaired interpersonal relationships.

Seclusion—A treatment modality in which the patient is placed in a safe, controlled, and secure environment that has a marked decrease in external stimuli.

Secondary gain—Benefits or attention that a patient receives from exhibiting certain behavior, from illness or from hospital admission, that are not direct consequences of that behavior.

Self-esteem—The degree to which an individual feels valued, competent, and worthwhile.

Somatization—An individual's reacting to psychological stressors and conflicts with physical symptoms.

Splitting—A primitive defense mechanism in which persons possessing a natural mix of both positive and negative attributes are perceived either "all good" or "all bad."

Substance abuse—The use of a psychoactive or mood-altering drug in a manner that includes a pattern of pathological use, impairment in occupational or social functioning, and a brief duration of at least one month.

Substance dependence—A compulsion to use a psychoactive or mood-altering drug, loss of control over the amount used, and continued use despite adverse consequences. Dependence occurs when tolerance to the drug develops, when withdrawal symptoms occur if the drug is not taken, and when the drug has been used for at least one month.

Suicidal ideation—Thoughts of taking one's own life.

Tardive dyskinesia—A disorder characterized by involuntary facial, tongue, and jaw movements resulting in bizarre grimacing, lip-smacking, and protrusion of the tongue. It can occur after years of treatment with neuroleptic drugs.

Tolerance—A decreasing response to repeated constant doses of a drug and/or the need for increasing doses to maintain a constant response.

Torticollis—A contracted state of the cervical muscles producing twisting of the neck and an unnatural position of the head.

Transference—The unconscious tendency to assign to others in one's present environment feelings and attitudes associated with significant others in one's early life. This usually refers to the patient's transfer to his therapist of feelings and attitudes associated with his parent. See *Countertransference.*

Underfunctioning (family member)—An adaptive family member who allows the dominant spouse or individual to make all decisions for the two of them. Harmony is maintained by the adaptive person. See *Overfunctioning.*

Index

Note: Numbers in *italic* refer to illustrations; numbers followed by *t* indicate tables.

Manual of PSYCHOSOCIAL NURSING INTERVENTIONS

Promoting Mental Health in Medical–Surgical Settings

Susan Lewis, M.A., R.N., C.S., Ph.D.
Ruth Dailey Knowles Grainger, Ph.D., A.R.N.P., C.S.
William A McDowell, Ph.D.
Robert J Gregory, Ph.D.
Roberta L Messner, R.N., M.S.N., C.I.C.

Here's an easy-to-use handbook on the psychosocial care of patients in the medical–surgical setting—both those with a psychiatric diagnosis and those under the normal stresses of physical illness and hospitalization. It provides the SPECIFIC step-by-step guidelines you need for effective planning and intervention! You'll find sound advice on helping clients with depression, post-traumatic stress disorders and other psychiatric disorders • addictive behaviors • chemical dependencies • and much more!

You'll also appreciate the insightful discussions on areas affecting your work, including legal issues . . . spiritual issues . . . psychotropic medications . . . and the family.

Plus . . . MANUAL OF PSYCHOSOCIAL INTERVENTIONS is designed for your convenience. The outline format is easy to read. The guidelines are practical, clear, and based on a nursing process approach. And the material is presented on a level consistent with your background. It's an effective tool when caring for medical–surgical clients!

W.B. SAUNDERS COMPANY
Harcourt Brace Jovanovich, Inc.

ISBN 0-7216-5763-X